Implementing School-Based Occupational Therapy Services

This book focuses on providing occupational therapy sensory interventions through a tiered approach to help improve academic participation, covering assessment of the sensory aspects of the environment and population, as well as at the group level.

Chapters showcase how occupational therapy practitioners can effectively contribute to each tier of the multi-tiered system of supports (MTSS) framework, with an emphasis on Tiers 1 and 2. The book also provides evidence-based methods to monitor outcomes of provided interventions and discuss how and when to modify the interventions, and highlights innovative strategies to support a broad range of students, especially those who may need additional assistance but do not qualify for specialized services.

While there are many reasons students might require support, this book zeroes in on sensory processing challenges and their impact on classroom participation and academic performance. By addressing these needs, occupational therapy practitioners can foster a more inclusive, engaging, and supportive learning environment for every student.

Aimee Piller PhD, OTR/L, BCP, FAOTA, is the owner and director of Piller Child Development, an outpatient pediatric therapy company with three locations in the greater Phoenix area. She is a practicing occupational therapist with almost 20 years of experience in a variety of pediatric settings including outpatient home health and schools.

"A must-read for anyone in the school setting, *Implementing School-Based Occupational Therapy Services: A Multi-Tiered Approach to Sensory Processing Needs* offers practical strategies to address sensory challenges. Dr. Piller combines research-based insights with real-world applications, making complex concepts accessible. This book empowers occupational therapy practitioners to support all children, fostering inclusive classrooms and promoting independence. Informative and inspiring, it's an essential resource for school personnel."

> **Lauren Andelin, OTD, OTR/L, BCP,** *Assistant Professor of Occupational Therapy at Virginia Commonwealth University.*

"This is a must read for all school-based occupational therapists and should be required reading in occupational therapy pediatric coursework. Gone are the days of occupational therapists solely providing direct fine motor interventions in the school setting. Occupational therapy must be prepared to provide all forms of occupational therapy to address academic, behavioral, and social-emotional needs under a multi-tiered system and this book provides a guideline for how to implement such strategies. It provides the necessary background to understand the need for providing appropriate services, how to evaluate for services, and usable strategies to implement at each level. The author clearly has strong knowledge of sensory-based approaches and how to implement them in the school setting."

> **Jessica McHugh Conlin, PhD, OTR/L, BCP, OT** *with 25 years of experience in school-based practice.*

Implementing School-Based Occupational Therapy Services

A Multi-Tiered Approach to Sensory Processing Needs

Aimee Piller

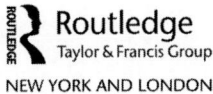

Routledge
Taylor & Francis Group

NEW YORK AND LONDON

Designed cover image: Getty Images

First published 2026
by Routledge
605 Third Avenue, New York, NY 10158

and by Routledge
4 Park Square, Milton Park, Abingdon, Oxon, OX14 4RN

Routledge is an imprint of the Taylor & Francis Group, an informa business

ISBN: 978-1-032-65475-1 (hbk)
ISBN: 978-1-032-65474-4 (pbk)
ISBN: 978-1-032-65476-8 (ebk)

DOI: 10.4324/9781032654768

Typeset in Times New Roman
by Deanta Global Publishing Services, Chennai, India

To access the support material please visit: www.routledge.com/9781032654744

Contents

Introduction   1

1   A Brief Review of Legislation Guiding School-Based
    Occupational Therapy Practice   5

2   Sensory Processing and Its Impact on Education   30

3   Multi-Tiered System of Supports and Occupational
    Therapy and Sensory Needs   50

4   Assessing the Need for Sensory Interventions   78

5   Designing Interventions to Address Sensory
    Processing Needs   115

6   Evaluating Outcomes of Interventions   156

7   Working with a Multidisciplinary Team   179

8   Changing the Service Model: Facilitating Lasting Change   204

    Index   *223*

Introduction

I became an occupational therapist in 2006. Wide-eyed, armed with a master's degree in occupational therapy and a bachelor's degree in elementary education, I was on my way to work in schools. I loved education, and I loved even more the idea of helping children who struggled with mainstream education thrive and grow. Working as an occupational therapist in a school setting was my dream, and I could not wait to work with teachers, parents, and especially with students.

My first job was in early childhood education at a local public school with a solid reputation for providing high-quality special education services. In fact, many families moved into the district specifically to access these special education services for their children. I was the only occupational therapist working in the early childhood age group, but the district had a team that consisted of one occupational therapist and four occupational therapy assistants. While I served different students, this committed occupational therapy team met every week to collaborate and ensure continuity from preschool through to high school. Looking back, perhaps my ignorance was my best asset. I did not know how the previous therapist had done things at the school. I had no prior experience working as an occupational therapist in a school setting. And I had done my internships in medical settings, so my only reference for schools was from my own educational background. As a young therapist, I was eager to learn and grow. I attended the team meetings each week, even though these were unpaid. I wanted to be part of the team and ensure I knew what was happening with the students and staff. Meeting with the teachers, speech-language pathologists, and other team members allowed me to develop a sense of camaraderie with my colleagues, building my confidence and giving me a feeling of fulfillment.

It was a learning curve, to say the least. I worked hard to understand the student's needs, learn the flow of the day, and understand the special education processes, all while learning to be an occupational therapist. I loved that job and loved my team. Had I not moved across the country a few years later, I would probably still be working there today.

Perhaps it was because I did not know anything different, but I ended up developing a method to implement occupational therapy services using a tiered

DOI: 10.4324/9781032654768-1

approach. In a way, I provided services in a multi-tiered system of supports (MTSS) long before MTSS was law. The district was very supportive of therapy, which meant I could see almost every student in my caseload for at least 60 minutes a week under their Individualized Education Plan (IEP). This was great for the students, but with only one therapist working four days a week, my schedule quickly became full. I had to develop a better method to meet the service minute requirements and ensure students received high-quality care.

Once a week, I would pull the students out of class to my occupational therapy area and provide very traditional occupational therapy services, working with either one or two students who shared similar goals. As my caseload grew, I became creative with how to best use my time. There was one teacher I worked with closely who was welcoming of my expertise and suggestions, and I asked her if I could come in once a week and run an occupational therapy group focused on motor and sensory needs. She agreed since, while I was running the class, she could either work individually with a student on their goals or plan other lessons. I offered services designed to address the student's goals on my caseload, but all students in the classroom benefited from the occupational therapy group time.

The model proved successful, and other teachers asked me to come in and run an occupational therapy group once or twice a week in their classrooms. This was great for me. I could continue providing highly individualized services to the students on my caseload while also serving other students. I balanced my workload by providing group therapy once a week instead of individual treatment for every service minute. This helped me use my time more efficiently and allowed me the time to service clients one-on-one.

The teachers observed the impact of sensory interventions on their students' success and wanted to provide even more sensory support. Every teacher that year advocated for sensory equipment in their teaching classroom and asked for my input on how to spend their supply budget on these sensory tools. They also saw the value of providing sensory input throughout the day but recognized this required time from classroom staff. The teachers got together as a team and advocated for the administration to provide an additional classroom assistant who reported to me, the occupational therapist. This person's main job was to ensure sensory diets (specified sensory accommodations to meet a student's sensory needs) were implemented according to how I prescribed them, and to work with me to ensure the student's sensory needs were met. The teachers continued to welcome me in their classrooms and wanted my suggestions because they recognized that my support helped their students succeed.

Little did I know, all those years ago, that experience would be the foundation for this book. I implemented Tier 1 and Tier 2 interventions before the idea of MTSS, and I saw the effectiveness of these interventions. So did the teachers. One aftermath of the COVID pandemic is that more and more children have increased sensory needs. There are so many students, and there are not enough practitioners to service them all.

That is why I have written this book. Based on my experience in implementing this model, much like MTSS, I want to share and help occupational therapy practitioners, teachers, and administrators see the value of occupational therapy as a regular element of the classroom, interwoven throughout the school day.

In short, this book will demonstrate how to implement and examine occupational therapy services in the school system under the tiered model. The Every Student Succeeds Act (ESSA) of 2015 outlines the requirements of schools to provide support for all students under an MTSS framework to facilitate academic, behavioral, and social-emotional well-being. Occupational therapists have traditionally practiced under what is now considered Tier 3 of MTSS, providing direct services to individuals who qualified for special education services. However, occupational therapy practitioners have much to offer all students school-wide. This book outlines how occupational therapy practitioners can provide school-based services at each tier (with a particular focus on Tier 1 and Tier 2) to service all students who may need support. While students may be identified as needing support for a variety of reasons, this book will focus on sensory processing to support classroom participation and academic-related occupational performance.

In the first part of this book, I will provide an overview of relevant laws that guide occupational therapy services in the educational system. I will then move to look at how each tier can specifically relate to occupational therapy services and sensory processing needs. Since Tier 3 is considered traditional for occupational therapy services and most practitioners are well-versed in providing this support, I will emphasize and discuss the importance of assessment and intervention at Tier 1 and Tier 2. From here, I will look at how occupational therapy practitioners can implement high-quality interventions at each tier that fit within the occupational therapy framework rather than just sensory suggestions that anyone can provide.

But, why should we focus on implementing services at Tier 1 and Tier 2 levels? As occupational therapists and school personnel, it helps us support more students and moves us from a caseload model to a workload model, decreasing stress and burnout. Due to the high caseloads of therapists, freeing up more time to focus on individuals with higher or more specific needs will benefit everyone. For each of the tiers, I will outline specific evaluation methods, develop treatment plans and interventions, and monitor outcomes to ensure interventions are meeting the goals of ESSA. These will specifically relate to sensory processing needs in the school setting, as this is one of the most common reasons students are referred to occupational therapy services. Finally, I will provide a guide on advocating for occupational therapy interventions at Tier 1 and Tier 2, and offer methods to work with and train school personnel to implement a successful program in the school setting.

Occupational therapy has so much to offer our clients and the educational system. Yet, if we continue to service every client under an individualized model, not only will some students be neglected and miss out on services, but occupational practitioners will become burnt out. They may leave the school setting or, worse, leave the profession. With a slight shift in thinking, occupational therapy has the potential to impact all students, while allowing practitioners to reserve our time for those who have higher needs. When we work with teachers, administrators, and school personnel through an MTSS model, occupational therapy can change the field of education and help ensure success for all students. Occupational therapy can become so much more than just a related service provider – we can become an essential part of the education system.

Chapter 1

A Brief Review of Legislation Guiding School-Based Occupational Therapy Practice

Legislation Guiding School-Based Occupational Therapy Practice

In public education, legislation at the federal level guides the implementation and funding of occupational therapy services. Therefore, it is essential that occupational therapy practitioners understand these laws and regulations as they directly impact their practice and the occupational therapy services available in their school settings. In this chapter, we will firstly review the history of occupational therapy in school settings and examine the changes in legislation that guide our practice today. We will then examine the role and responsibility of occupational therapists in creating an inclusive learning environment for all students, supporting students and staff in ensuring everyone has access to education regardless of their sensory or additional needs.

A Short History of Occupational Therapy in Public Education

Before the 1960s, the role of the occupational therapist working within the school system was rare. Unfortunately, this meant that many students with accessibility needs were often excluded or restricted from benefiting from the same level of education as their peers. However, beginning with the Civil Rights movement, the 1960s and 1970s brought about many changes in the United States of America that led to new legislation that ensured equal access to education for many underserved and underrepresented populations. These changes included making public schools accessible to children with disabilities.

Prior to 1975, children with disabilities were often denied access to public education, and some states even had laws prohibiting students with disabilities from attending public school (U.S. Department of Education, 2024). Instead, they may have been sent to special schools, placed in hospitals for children with disabilities, or institutionalized, leaving few children with disabilities to be educated in the public-school setting. While some of these institutions included education for the basic academic skills of reading, writing, and math, the focus

DOI: 10.4324/9781032654768-2

was on vocational skills building (Rioux & Chandler, 2019). These settings may have had occupational therapists working with the students, but this was not a requirement and often institutions did not have occupational therapists available.

It was not until 1975 that Congress passed the Education for All Handicapped Children Act (EHA) (Public Law 94–142) to ensure that all children had access to public education. This was the precursor to the Individuals with Disabilities Education Act (IDEA), which now guides the provision of occupational therapy services in the school setting and makes offering occupational therapy services a requirement for schools (Coates, 1985). As occupational therapists, it is important to look back at the history and contents of these legislations to understand the significance of our role within the school setting, inspiring us to strive for continuous change. Let us review these past laws to reflect on their impact in our work today.

Individuals with Disabilities Education Act (1975)

Originally known as the Education for All Handicapped Children Act (EHA) (Public Law 94–142), the Individuals with Disabilities Act (IDA) was implemented in 1975. This law aimed to ensure that every state was required to offer public education to all children, regardless of disability status. Before the implementation of EHA, nearly two million children were excluded from receiving an education, making this new legislation hugely impactful. One of the primary focuses of this law was to protect the rights of children and families, meaning that it was the responsibility of the state to identify and meet the needs of children with disabilities. The state, and consequently schools, were encouraged to support and improve the results and outcomes of children from birth through to graduation, and to guide them in their transition beyond school into their young adult lives (U.S. Department of Education, 2024).

In 1990, the United States Congress passed an amendment that expanded EHA, known as the Individuals with Disabilities Education Act (IDEA). This law addressed early intervention, specialized instruction, and related services. The major difference between EHA and IDEA was an expansion of who was eligible for special education services. IDEA also included additional age groups beyond school-age children, including infants and toddlers. Further, IDEA focused on keeping children in their neighborhood schools rather than requiring them to travel to schools far from their homes, and it required that children with disabilities were educated in the least restrictive environment (LRE), ensuring access to non-disabled peers (U.S. Department of Education, 2024).

Under this new law, occupational therapy was identified as a required related service to support students with disabilities in their access to and participation in special education services. IDEA differentiates occupational therapy from special education services but includes it as a requirement. Despite EHA allowing all children with disabilities to access public education, many students were still excluded from a range of education services. The implementation of IDEA helped resolve these issues. Consequently, the changes in the law meant that schools had to increase their education services to include children with disabilities.

The immense impact of both EHA and IDEA on children within the US school system cannot be understated. With the addition of EHA and IDEA, more than 7.5 million children could access educational services and other services to increase functional outcomes and results in preparation for adult life. The statistics speak for themselves: after the implementation of IDEA, graduation rates and postsecondary education enrollment increased nationally (Rioux & Chandler, 2019; U.S. Department of Education, 2024).

Now, let us dive deeper into what IDEA states and stands for. By understanding this legislation fully, we will be able to frame our role as occupational therapists in the school setting, reminding us of the key principles to consider when working with the young people we encounter.

Individuals with Disabilities Education Act (IDEA)

IDEA is divided into four parts.

- **Part A**: Outlines the importance of providing education for all students, specifically focusing on ensuring those with disabilities are given the same rights as all other children.
- **Part B**: Outlines how these services should be implemented for school-aged children.
- **Part C**: Outlines the early intervention services aimed at children from birth through to two years of age.
- **Part D**: Outlines federal grant funding and supports the education of students with disabilities.

We will now explore each of the first three parts of IDEA in depth, explaining how this law should impact the practice of occupational therapy in the school setting (U.S. Department of Education, 2019).

PART A

Part A outlines the importance of providing education for all students, specifically focusing on ensuring those with disabilities are given the same rights as all other children. This means all children have the right to a "free and appropriate education," also known as FAPE (Rioux & Chandler, 2019).

There are a few key aspects to consider when dealing with IDEA and FAPE. First, the family is an integral part of the educational team. They are required to be included in their child's educational process, and educational teams must work with parents and caregivers to ensure their needs are heard, understood, and addressed. Secondly, whole school approaches should be developed to ensure that all children can access the provided education and curriculums. In addition to general education and curriculums, the school must provide individualized, specialized instruction when needed. This means that schools need to take an inclusive approach to education and focus on implementing instructional methods designed for various learning styles and needs.

Education is typically managed at the local school district level, with guidelines provided by individual states. However, IDEA is clear that state and local school districts must implement services under IDEA, with the federal government providing assistance and guidance in implementing the provisions outlined by the law. Therefore, each school district is responsible for ensuring their school meets the requirements for servicing all students, regardless of disability, in compliance with federal law. Children must have an identified disability that impacts their access to education from peers of the same age in order to be eligible for services under IDEA.

Eligibility Categories According to IDEA   There are 14 different eligibility categories in IDEA for special education services, which are classified as low-incidence, medium-incidence, and high-incidence disabilities. Table 1.1 details these, including a summary of each eligibility criteria.

PART B

Part B of IDEA addresses how schools should implement the assistance offered to children with disabilities, ensuring that the education provided in the school environment is accessible to all.

In accordance with Part A of IDEA, the full law allocates funds for a variety of services that children may need to access education, including requirements for staff and the individualized education program (IEP). Within IDEA, procedures are outlined that indicate the rights of parents should they be in disagreement with the IEP team, including procedural safeguards, mediation, due process, and appeals. Importantly, parents have a right to seek an outside independent educational evaluation (IEE).

IEEs may occur in any area that is tested, including occupational therapy. Occupational therapists working outside of schools may perform in IEEs and provide recommendations related to education when evaluating children through this method. If occupational therapists who work in private practice perform IEEs, they must have an understanding of the laws and requirements of occupational therapy services at the federal, state, and district levels, which may differ significantly from the medical model requirements in the private outpatient therapy setting. In a school setting, the IEE becomes part of the student's school

Table 1.1 Categories of Special Education with Incidence Level (U.S. Department of Education, 2019)

Category	Incidence Level	Summary of Eligibility Criteria
Hearing impaired	Low	Includes conductive and sensorineural loss Measured in terms of decibels Varies by state
Deafness	Low	Unaided minimum, pure tone average 66–70dB
Visual impairment (including blindness)	Low	Based on visual acuity and visual field Varies by state
Deaf-blindness	Low	Meets criteria for hearing impairment and visual impairment
Orthopedic impairment	Low	Orthopedic impairment caused by congenital anomalies, disease, or other causes Evidence of severe orthopedic impairment, motor impairment with deficits in quality, speed, or accuracy by at least two standard deviations in fine motor, gross motor, or self-help; condition is permanent (longer than 60 days)
Traumatic brain injury	Low	Nonspecific and varies by state
Multiple disabilities	Low	Varies by state based on a combination of disabilities and severity
Autism	Medium	Impairments in social interaction and communication, restricted, repetitive, or stereotyped patterns of behavior
Developmental delay	Medium	Delay in one or more of the following areas: cognitive development, physical/motor development, communication development, social/emotional development, and adaptive development; varies across states as to severity
Intellectual disability	Medium	Subaverage intellectual functioning and adaptive functioning; severity can vary by state, but generally should be at least two standard deviations below the mean
Emotional disturbance	Medium	Serious behavior problems that are present over a long period of time (typically more than six months); specificity and severity varies by state
Specific learning disability	High	Varies by state, but is often based on data from Response to Intervention (RTI); discrepancy is present between intellectual ability and achievement (often at least 1.5 standard deviations below the mean)
Speech language impairment	High	Includes articulation, voice, fluency, and language disorders; varies by state, but is typically based on standardized, norm-referenced assessments
Other health impairment	High	Acute health problems that result in limitations to strength, vitality, and limited or heightened alertness to the environment; includes attention-deficit disorder (ADD) and attention-deficit/hyperactivity disorder (ADHD)

record and evaluation report, and the IEP team has to consider its outcomes. However, the IEP team does not have to accept the results and recommendations.

Table 1.2 below outlines the required components of the IEP, highlighting which areas are the responsibility of the occupational therapist within the program. These components are there to support the student needing individualized assistance to meet their goals.

Whilst focused on public education, Part B also allows students who attend private schools or are home schooled to access services through their local school districts. Child find is a program that helps to identify children who may

Table 1.2 Required Components in IEP

Component	Brief Description	Occupational Therapist May be Responsible for Portions
Statement of present levels of academic achievement and functional performance	Includes how disability may impact participation in general education	Yes
Measurable annual goals	Academic and functional goals that address the child's needs Benchmark short-term objectives outline steps to meet goals	Yes
Progress reporting	Summary of child's progress towards goals and how progress will be measured	Yes
Statement of special education, related services, and supplemental aids and services	Includes services the child will receive and when those will begin	Yes
Statement of modifications or supports	Description of modifications or supports provided to the student to facilitate progress toward goals	Yes
Explanation of the extent to which the student will participate in the general education classroom	Amount of time the child will participate with nondisabled peers	May make recommendations
Individual accommodations	Accommodations needed to measure performance and achievement	May make recommendations
Transition services and post-secondary goals	Required for students at age 16	Yes

have disabilities and may need specialized instructions (U.S. Department of Education, 2017a). Many community organizations, local educational agencies, state educational agencies, and early intervention programs assist with Child find. In addition, private medical providers, including occupational therapists, may also refer children to a local school district for evaluation. This helps to ensure that even children who do not attend a local public school can access services under IDEA.

Another important aspect of Part B is the provision of transitional services to help students progress to adulthood and post-graduation. These services must be in the IEP by the time the student reaches 16, and the student should be part of the planning and goal-setting process for transition services (U.S. Department of Education, 2020).

Finally, a fundamental aspect of IDEA is that children should be educated in the least restrictive environment (LRE), meaning that students who have disabilities should spend as much time in the general education classroom with nondisabled peers as possible. The LRE allows students to engage with peers socially, establish peer role models, and help students prepare for life in the community. In addition, nondisabled peers also have an opportunity to connect with students with disabilities, promoting community and acceptance. In these situations, support can, and should be, provided in the general education setting to help students participate. Services, including occupational therapy, should also strive for LRE when providing services to support learning and participation within the classroom with peers.

Typically the LRE is where students with disabilities spend time in classrooms and other spaces with students without disabilities, but the LRE must be considered on an individual basis, which is determined by the IEP team (Schneider & Chandler, 2019). Some students with sensory processing differences may have difficulties with auditory and tactile sensitivities. The busy mainstream classroom may actually be more restrictive, due to their sensory processing, than a smaller, more individualized classroom. Therefore, it is important to consider each student's needs, rather than just considering the general education setting as the LRE.

PART C

Part C of IDEA outlines the services for children from birth until their third birthday, often known as early intervention services. Once a child becomes three years old, they move to Part B of IDEA. One of the main goals of this portion of IDEA is to set children up for success early, maximizing their potential, helping families meet their children's needs, and reducing the costs of special education and related services later down the line.

Part C uses a multidisciplinary approach when evaluating which services are required to meet the diverse needs of infants and young children. The intervention approach is family-centered for both the evaluation and intervention planning, and it emphasizes a coaching model to help caregivers learn to implement strategies provided to them by professionals. The services for children receiving treatment under Part C of IDEA are outlined in an Individualized Family Service Plan (IFSP), and these services aim to address specific needs in physical, cognitive, communication, social/emotional, and adaptive development (U.S. Department of Education, 2019).

Some components of the IFSP include the following.

- The child and family demographic, health, and social information, including details on what the transition will look like when the child turns three years of age.
- The functional abilities of the child, summarizing present development levels, including hearing, vision, physical health, strengths, and needs. This section also includes a summary of functional abilities in social-emotional skills (positive social-emotional skills), cognition (acquiring and using knowledge and skills), and adaptive skills (taking appropriate actions to meet needs).
- An outline of the family and child's routines, including self-care, play, and sleep.
- Information on the service coordinator, as well as identified goals and additional resources available to the family. These goals should be developed in collaboration with the parents.
- Activities, procedures, and services that should be implemented to achieve goals.

(U.S. Department of Education, 2019)

REAUTHORIZATION OF IDEA (2004)

IDEA brought about incredible changes for students across the country, but more updates and adaptations were required. Congress reauthorized IDEA in 2004 with many expansions to the current law to meet the needs of students and to align with other federal laws, such as the No Child Left Behind Act, 20 U.S.C. § 6319 (2002). Some of the main additions included early intervening services and increased standards and accountability. Early intervening services are an essential component of this expansion as they provide services and support to children who may not have been previously identified under special education services (U.S. Department of Education, 2024).

However, more change was to come with the Every Student Succeeds Act over a decade later, which continues to directly inform our practice as occupational therapists in school settings.

Every Student Succeeds Act (ESSA, 2015)

The Every Student Succeeds Act (ESSA) was signed into law in 2015. It was written to support and advocate for the success of all students in school settings. It focused on supporting equity in education, protecting disadvantaged students and those with high needs. To achieve this, it offered support for expanding preschool programs as well as additional funding for low-income students, promoting high academic standards and statewide assessment requirements (U.S. Department of Education, n.d.). One important aspect of ESSA is that specialized instructional support personnel, including occupational therapists, must be involved in program development and the implementation of accommodations (Schneider & Chandler, 2019). ESSA requires the development and monitoring of goals through progress monitoring, but it allows the districts to develop their own goals and ways to monitor progress (Cahill, 2019). One way this can be achieved in ESSA is through Response to Intervention (RTI).

Response to Intervention (RTI)

Response to Intervention is designed to assist students before they reach a level of failure. Based on the student's needs, it provides high-quality instruction that is more individualized than the general curriculum, allowing the student to receive support that is specific to their areas of difficulty. Response to Intervention goes hand-in-hand with Positive Behavioral Support (PBS) to assist learning and behavior within the school setting.

With RTI and PBS, interprofessional teams work together to develop evidence-based interventions to support the student. To begin, the team has to identify and describe the student's academic and behavioral performance. This enables the team to effectively analyze areas of difficulty and establish a baseline of the student's performance. Over a period of time, several team members gather data at different points throughout the school day and week, helping them to develop a hypothesis as to why there is a concern for the student. From these results, the team identifies a specific performance or behavior to monitor, and they develop an intervention plan to address this based on the hypothesis that was previously formulated. Once the plan is executed, it is monitored to determine if it should be continued, changed, or discontinued (Cahill, 2019). In Chapter 6, we will explore progress monitoring and monitoring outcomes in more detail, but let us now turn to the latest part of ESSA: the multi-tiered system of supports (MTSS).

Multi-Tiered System of Supports (MTSS)

The multi-tiered system of supports (MTSS) is part of ESSA that took full effect during the 2017–2018 school year. In contrast to previous legislation and assistance offered, MTSS allows for all students to benefit from support through a tiered system, which is factored based on their specific needs. In addition to this, MTSS provides not just academic support to students, but also both social and emotional support (Walker et al., 2023).

Similar to RTI, MTSS is an interprofessional model where a team of school personnel work together to find solutions that support students towards success. However, another key difference is that it expands the RTI model by seeking to provide services and support through what is known as early intervening services. Previously, in order to qualify for special education services, students often had to exhibit a delay that is well below their expected grade level. In MTSS, the goal is to support a student before they are at a point of failure, and a huge benefit of MTSS is that it can be provided to students in the general education model. By providing support early, rather than waiting for students to fail, the hope is that more students will be successful in the general education model and not need higher intensity, specialized instruction.

Members of the MTSS team include teachers, speech-language pathologists, occupational therapists, physical therapists, psychologists and counselors, and many other school personnel. The team works together to identify problems, suggest solutions, develop and implement a plan for the student, and evaluate its effectiveness. Key components of MTSS are universal screening of all students to identify those who may need additional support, evidence-based interventions, and systematic data collection for progress monitoring. Three tiers are considered under this model, which we will now outline and define.

Tier 1 interventions are universal learning supports that are classroom-wide, encompassing the needs of around 80% of students in the school, but are interventions provided to all students. The interventions are designed to be preventative and proactive to support students at all levels, including those identified as needing specialized instruction. Interventions such as universal learning designs fall under Tier 1.

Tier 2 interventions are targeted group interventions, which can apply to approximately 10–15% of students. These students have been identified through universal screenings as potentially being at risk of falling behind. The interventions are targeted at specific needs through a small group model, with the small group's needs being fairly cohesive. For example, students who struggle with attention and have identified sensory processing needs may be placed into a group model for intervention separate from a small group of students who were identified as being at risk for falling behind in math. Interventions focus on the child's strengths and help to provide support for potential areas of concern. Therefore, students in the group who were identified as having attention difficulties due to sensory processing needs would have interventions targeted at sensory processing, tailored to the group needs, with the goal of improving attention in the classroom. The group identified as having difficulties in math would receive interventions designed to improve math skills. While the same

Table 1.3 Multi-Tiered System of Supports (MTSS)

Tier Level	Description	Components (American Institute for Research [AIR], 2024)	Role of Occupational Therapist (Piller et al., 2023)
Tier 1	Universal/core instruction	Evidence and research-based Problem-solving teams Universal screening Progress monitoring Professional development	Training and education for teachers Universal screenings Modifications to the school environment Population-based interventions
Tier 2	Small group targeted interventions	More intensive Small groups Differentiated instruction	Design and monitoring of group interventions Episodic problem-solving with staff
Tier 3	Intensive intervention	Individualized and group Connections to community agencies	Direct and consultative services typically under an IEP

(Cahill, 2019; Walker et al., 2023; Piller et al., 2023)

students may be in both groups, goals and activities during the group time would be very different to address the needs of the group they are currently in.

Tier 3 interventions are offered to students under IDEA when a student has been identified as needing individualized and intensive support. This is a small percentage of students, less than 5% of the general population within a school setting (American Occupational Therapy Association [AOTA], 2012; Cahill, 2019). The specifics of each tier will be addressed further in Chapter 3, but Table 1.3 summarizes each tier for reference below.

Other Important Legislations and Considerations for School-Based Practice

Outside of the school setting, the majority of occupational therapy services are provided under a medical model. School-based practitioners have a unique role in providing educationally relevant occupational therapy services. However, in many school districts, occupational therapy services are still covered by Medicaid funds. Therefore, the occupational therapy practitioner must provide documentation that meets the guidelines of both the school setting (often district-dependent) and state Medicaid requirements.

FAMILY EDUCATIONAL RIGHTS AND PRIVACY ACT (FERPA)/ HEALTH INSURANCE AND PORTABILITY AND ACCOUNTABILITY ACT (HIPAA)

In educational settings, the Family Educational Rights and Privacy Act of 1974 (FERPA) 20 U.S.C. § 1232g (1974) protects the rights and privacy of students

Table 1.4 Comparison of IEP and 504 Plan

IEP	504
IDEA	Rehabilitation Act
Specialized instruction	Accommodations
What a student learns	How a student learns
Must fall into one of the eligibility categories	Any disability

and their families. This law protects the privacy of records for all students under IDEA. Since occupational therapy is often billed to Medicaid in the school setting, therapists must also adhere to the privacy guidelines of the Health Insurance and Portability and Accountability Act (HIPAA) of 1996, Pub. L. No. 104–191 (1996). Occupational therapy practitioners working in school settings must be familiar with both FERPA and HIPAA guidelines when it comes to the privacy and confidentiality of students and records (AOTA, 2017).

SECTION 504

Section 504, 29 U. S. C. § 794 (1973) is part of the Rehabilitation Act Amendments of 2004 under the Americans with Disability Act of 2008. This law was designed to prevent discrimination due to having a disability and promote equal access for all. Equal access also applies to the education setting. The funding for Section 504 does not come from the same funds as those reserved for IDEA, and students may qualify for a 504 Plan based on any disability, not just those outlined under IDEA. The primary purpose of a 504 Plan is to provide equal access for students with disabilities and include environmental adaptations and reasonable accommodations. In some districts, occupational therapy services may be provided under a 504 Plan. This plan frequently outlines supports (including sensory supports and accommodations) in many districts.

Now we have explored how occupational therapy came to be in schools, let us dive deeper into how this legislation guides our practice in creating inclusive and accessible learning environments.

Occupational Therapy as a Related Service

As mentioned earlier in the chapter, the introduction of IDEA led to occupational therapy being classed as a related service within the school system. Related services are defined as "transportation and such developmental, corrective and other supportive services [that] are required to assist a child with a disability to benefit from special education" (U.S Department of Education, 2017b), with other related services include counseling services, psychological services, and some medical services (U.S. Department of Education, 2017a).

This impacts the role and opportunities of the occupational therapy practitioner in the school setting (Rioux & Chandler, 2019). Occupational therapy practitioners are frequently considered noncertified personnel and often fall under different benefit categories than certified personnel (i.e. teachers, speech-language pathologists, etc.). This can impact what occupational therapy practitioners qualify for in programs, such as state retirement programs, and other benefits, including certain positions held within the school system. As occupational therapy is a related service, occupational therapy practitioners are not typically required to carry a separate certification, such as a teaching endorsement or license, to work in the school setting. This differs from speech-language pathologists, who are typically required to carry this certification in most states. As a result, occupational therapists do not often serve as the team lead or case manager on an IEP. However, there are allowances for occupational therapists to serve as the case manager under the MTSS framework (Cahill, 2019). In addition, a child must qualify for special education under one of the 14 categories to receive occupational therapy services under IDEA, meaning that meeting the criteria for occupational therapy services is not enough to warrant occupational therapy services.

It is essential to understand that, as a related service, occupational therapists are in place to support the current service and educational model that exists within the school setting. The occupational therapy practitioner should support the academic curriculum and other services provided to the student in the school. In some school settings, occupational therapy has no separate goals. Rather, the occupational therapy practitioner supports all of the goals in the IEP. This represents a true interprofessional occupational therapy model as a related service supporting the goals and services in the IEP. However, in other districts, occupational therapists provide their own measurable goals that support academics, such as a writing goal or sensory processing goal related to following directions.

Occupational Therapy Practitioner Scope of Practice in the School Setting

Occupational therapy practitioners are guided by laws governing special education services to provide educationally relevant services, meaning the services provided include support for the child's participation in the educational program (Rioux & Chandler, 2019). The occupational therapist is responsible for the occupational therapy process in the school setting, including evaluation, service coordinators and case managers, direct service providers, consultative and collaborative services providers within the IEP and educational team, trainer, advocate, and providing schoolwide systems of support (AOTA, 2017). Occupational therapy practitioners should follow the guidelines outlined in IDEA, state rules and regulations, and district guidelines regarding when and how these services are provided within their unique setting. District procedures guiding the implementation of occupational therapy may differ greatly between districts and the occupational therapy practitioner must be aware of the district's policies and procedures in addition to state and federal laws. However, when working in the school setting, the occupational therapy practitioner must remember two main limits to the scope of practice. First, all services provided must be in relation to education and access to education. If a student has identified needs that occupational therapy can support, but they are not related to educational access or participation, these lie outside the scope of practice of the occupational therapy practitioner in the school setting. Second, occupational therapy practitioners provide a related service meaning they are there to support the child's engagement and participation in education. Therefore, it is essential that the occupational therapy practitioner works closely with other school personnel to ensure they support the needs of the student to access and participate in educational activities.

Let us now take a look at the main aims occupational therapists should strive for when working in school settings, and how they can assist teachers in achieving these goals, such as providing inclusive education and working to offer a universal design for learning.

Inclusive Education

Inclusive education is a term that refers to supporting access for all students in all activities and environments. It is a worldwide initiative recognized by many countries as a basic human right (Wray et al., 2022). The term inclusive education goes beyond providing the LRE, as outlined in IDEA, to provide supportive environments and instructional methods that allow all students to access education. Historically, LRE has been the goal of education for children with disabilities with the intent to have placement, as outlined in the IEP, to be one of the main responsibilities of IEP teams. However, inclusive education is more extensive than LRE and seeks to provide a setting conducive to educating all students. Integration, rather than segregation, is the goal (Nilholm, 2020). Inclusivity is a concept that the profession of occupational therapy has held as a core value for people across its lifespan. Occupational therapy practitioners are skilled in helping to modify the environment and methods of instruction to help match the needs of the person, including individuals and groups. Providing support and consultation, as well as being a key team member in developing inclusive education plans, is within the scope and expertise of the occupational therapist working in the school setting.

Whilst inclusive education is the main goal, barriers do exist. Barriers to inclusive education include knowledge of how to identify and implement inclusive educational methods and environments, traditional reliance on a more segregated education model, and attitudes toward how educators view inclusive education (Nilholm, 2020). However, each of these barriers provides an opportunity for the occupational therapy practitioner to play a vital role in implementing inclusive education within the school setting. Occupational therapy practitioners can help address attitudinal and environmental barriers to inclusive education through training and support. In addition, occupational therapists can support teachers and other school personnel to help demonstrate the value of inclusivity for all students and staff involved. This will be explored further in later chapters.

Universal Design for Learning

Universal design for learning (UDL) is the expectation in public education. It encompasses the idea that all students should have access to educational opportunities by optimizing teaching and learning to fit the needs of diverse students. The ideas behind UDL are based on educational and neuropsychological theories about how people learn, and the goal of UDL is to accommodate all students, with the understanding that each student is unique and has diverse needs (Jimenez et al., 2007; Rose et al., 2005). Therefore, the focus is on providing multiple means of engagement, representation, and action and expression (Ralabate, 2011).

The concepts in UDL recognize the individuality of each student rather than approaching education from a one-size-fits-all model, or trying to make students conform to the general instructional method chosen by the teacher or district for all students. The goal is to make learning accessible for every student, including those with identified disabilities and those of various cultural backgrounds. Universal design for learning provides flexible learning environments, including physical and social environments that can accommodate different learning styles, levels of understanding, and need for support. Curriculums should be designed with adjustable education goals, teaching methods that can be easily modified, materials that can be customized to the learner's needs, and various methods to assess learning.

Teachers are well qualified to provide modifications to promote UDL within their teaching methods, and the occupational therapy practitioner can assist teachers in generating modifications to support neurodiverse students' needs. The teacher's expertise in pedagogy and the occupational therapy practitioner's expertise in task analysis and adaptation create a perfect collaborative team to ensure UDL is championed in the educational environment.

Let us explore the three main components of universal design for learning: engagement, representation, and action and expression (CAST, 2024).

ENGAGEMENT

The aim of engagement is to motivate students to learn by tapping into their interests and motivations, providing them with opportunities to engage fully in the learning process and experience feelings of success. As part of UDL, engagement includes ensuring the content and structure are sufficiently challenging to promote learning and growth, but not so difficult that students become frustrated or overwhelmed (CAST, 2024). The goal is to provide opportunities for students to engage in the learning process as a just-right challenge and experience feelings of success. As an occupational therapy practitioner in a school setting, it is important to understand and learn about a student's interests and involve them in the learning process through goal setting and gathering feedback from the student's perspective. This can be achieved through collaborative projects, providing individualized feedback, and offering a variety of options on how to complete assignments.

REPRESENTATION

The goal of representation is to give students various ways to acquire information and knowledge. Using a variety of mediums for instruction can provide students with opportunities to access information in different ways (CAST, 2024). Examples include videos, infographics, audiobooks, traditional textbooks, lectures, and hands-on learning activities. In addition, providing information in various languages and supplementing text with pictures can improve access for many students.

ACTION AND EXPRESSION

The goal of action and expression is to provide learners with different ways to demonstrate what they have learned (CAST, 2024). Traditionally, paper and pencil assessments have been the main learning assessment method. However, under UDL, teachers can provide a variety of opportunities and methods for students to demonstrate their knowledge on various topics, including oral and written methods, art projects, and digital media. Assistive technology is an essential part of action and expression and provides an excellent opportunity for the occupational therapist to provide support in this area.

NEURODIVERSITY-AFFIRMING EDUCATION

While not directly a part of UDL, neuro-affirming educational approaches take into consideration the diversity of neurological development and functioning that different students may have. Respecting and referring to the different ways student's brains work, neuro-affirming educational approaches value these differences and do not view one way of processing as better than another (Baumer & Frueh, 2021). Instead of viewing neurodiversity in individuals as something to be changed, it looks at these differences as a core part of human diversity, much like languages of different cultures. With a neurodiversity-affirming approach, teachers design classrooms, lessons, and routines to provide supportive environments that work towards a student's strengths, mainly considering the diverse neurological differences of those with autism, ADHD, dyslexia, and other learning differences. Teachers using a neuro-affirming approach to education respect neurodiversity, individualize learning to work towards a student's strengths, utilize strength-based and student-centered practices, and create an inclusive and supportive learning environment (Patten et al., 2024).

Occupational therapists, especially those practicing from a sensory integration and processing perspective, have always taken a neurodiversity-affirming approach to intervention. The original principles of Ayres Sensory Integration® are founded on principles of building on strengths, presenting "just right challenges", seeking client input and feedback on their goals, and maintaining a client-led individualized treatment session (Parham et al., 2011). Occupational therapists can assist teachers and other school personnel in developing and implementing a neuro-affirming approach to education by promoting strength-based educational strategies, developing methods to gather input and feedback from students of all ages and levels, and individualizing pedagogy through task analysis to meet the needs of diverse learners.

Occupational Therapy's Role in Developing Inclusive Education Settings

As the role of the occupational therapist is a related service by law, it is in their responsibilities and power to support teachers in developing an inclusive education setting. Since they are experts in task analysis, assessment, and evaluation, they are qualified to help design and modify environments, programs, and methods to meet the diverse needs of learners by working toward their strengths (AOTA, 2020).

For example, one important way the occupational therapist can promote inclusive education practices is to assess classroom tasks and routines. Assessment of the classroom routines can provide a glimpse into how routines and tasks support the needs of students, or how they may instead be a barrier to them. With this information, occupational therapy practitioners can modify and change the routine to fit the needs of diverse learners. In different ways, occupational therapy practitioners can work closely with teachers and paraprofessionals to provide modifications to instructional methods and grading of activities to increase or decrease the challenge of the activity through task analysis. This supports the UDL principle of engagement, and is something occupational therapy practitioners are accustomed to doing on an ongoing basis through the grading of activities to meet client needs.

In addition to the assessment and evaluation of classroom routines, an important role of the occupational therapy practitioner is to evaluate and modify the classroom environment to meet student needs as per the Person-Environment-Occupation theory (Law et al., 1996). Chapter 5 will explore in detail specific strategies on how to work with teachers when modifying their environments and activities, but the support and expertise of the occupational therapy practitioner can allow all students to access the curriculum without increasing the burden on the teacher. A full assessment of the physical features (such as seating options), social features (such as desk arrangement), and sensory features of the environment allows the occupational therapist to provide specialized recommendations to ensure a universal design for classrooms, promoting learning and independence rather than reliance on social supports.

Sensory Environment

As part of curating a neuro-affirming inclusive educational setting, the occupational therapist can provide assessments and modifications of the sensory environment, which can help increase the participation of all students and staff. To ensure the best fit between the environment, staff, and students, an occupational therapist can evaluate the criteria below in different classroom settings to promote accessible learning for all. While evidence on the effectiveness of sensory environmental modifications is still developing, the consideration of the sensory environment is important to help all students and staff access the school environment and feel safe and effective within that environment. Here are some general considerations of the sensory environment to consider in the school setting.

- **Visual environment**: Lighting, items on the wall, furniture arrangement, items on desks, colors of walls, carpet, etc.
- **Vestibular**: The openness of the space, proximity to walls, access to movement (variable seating options, places to stand or walk around, etc.).
- **Proprioception**: Access to fidgets, bands on chairs, etc.
- **Auditory**: Quiet spaces, noise-absorbing materials, proximity to others, and noise-dampening devices such as earplugs and headbands.
- **Tactile**: Access to tactile items such as weighted items and velcro on desks, and in areas such as reading corners (i.e. pillows, blankets, etc.).
- **Olfactory**: Calming scents, extraneous scents.

Along with the above criteria for assessing sensory environments, Figure 1.1 outlines an example of a classroom routines checklist that an occupational therapist may use to assess and evaluate the inclusivity of an education setting. It provides a data collection sheet that can be used to note daily classroom routines including the activity, such as "arriving in the classroom," a brief description of the main activities that occur during this time, the time (including the time of day and duration), and an area to note how the students and staff or teachers responded during this activity. This data can be shared with other school personnel to support any recommendations made to modify the learning environment.

Location of Observation:_____

Observer: _____   Date(s) of Observation: _____

Activity	Main Activities	Time	Reaction of Students	Reaction of Teacher/Staff
Entering Classroom Preparing for day	*Putting belongings away Preparing belongings for the day Getting settled into seats*	*10 minutes 8:15–8:25 AM*	*Approximately ¼ of students can follow the routine to put items away and be seated ready to work ¼ of students need assistance or cues from the teacher/classroom aide*	*The teacher provides visual and verbal cues to help students sequence tasks, gather materials, and prepare for the day*
Lesson One	Reading			
Lesson Two	Math			
Transition One				
Recess				
Transition Two				
Lunch				
Lesson Three				
Specials				

Additional Comments:

Figure 1.1 Classroom routines checklist. Image by author.

Occupational Therapy's Role in Changing Attitudes Toward Inclusive Education

Unfortunately, teachers, school administrators, and other school personnel may be resistant to modifying their current practices to create a more inclusive learning environment. Although these reasons may be understandable considering their working conditions, it is part of the occupational therapist's role to help support and modify these attitudes towards providing inclusive education.

Teachers may be reluctant to incorporate more inclusive measures into their teaching methods and environments because they feel unsupported or are unsure how to implement an inclusive model. Many teachers are already limited in terms of time due to the amount of work and requirements required to educate diverse students, and this may make them feel even more overwhelmed or stressed. Some educators may think that inclusive educational methods may increase their workload when these practices can greatly decrease it.

However, there are several ways occupational therapy practitioners can support teachers in making these changes to benefit all their students. For example, they can play an important role in training teachers and assisting them in setting up their classrooms early in the school year, helping them to promote inclusive learning. If the occupational therapy practitioner advocates for time to support teachers, this can decrease the burden on classroom teachers and have effects that last throughout the school year. In addition, training and working with classroom assistants is a key way to decrease the burden on teachers. When occupational therapy practitioners train classroom assistants, these essential classroom personnel can assist the teacher in ensuring that UDL principles are established in the classroom. They can work with the occupational therapy practitioner to monitor and modify routines, tasks, and the environment to ensure all students have access to learning without increasing the burden on the primary classroom teacher.

Additionally, administrators may initially be hesitant to provide time for occupational therapy practitioners to engage in evaluating, supporting, and training teachers to provide inclusive education. This is often due to the high cost of occupational therapy practitioners providing services for an increasing number of students with occupational therapy needs. Administrators may be reluctant to allow for time for occupational therapy practitioners to collaborate with teachers and classroom assistants because this may not be considered billable time under state Medicaid reimbursement, which is a main payment source for the occupational therapy practitioner in the school setting.

If that is the case, occupational therapy practitioners can gradually increase the teacher's and administrator's knowledge of the many aspects they can address beyond direct services. Rather than all teachers receiving occupational therapy support, the school could begin with just one teacher who is open to the idea. Another good starting point is the general education classroom, with many students receiving direct occupational therapy services under an IEP. Working closely with one teacher allows the occupational therapy practitioner to gather data through progress monitoring to support an inclusive model. In addition, the teacher can provide qualitative data on how the support of the occupational therapist decreased the burden on the teacher. Armed with data, the occupational therapist can present a more thought-out, data-informed proposal on how occupational therapy practitioners can support inclusive education at a school-wide level.

With this in mind, let us look at an example of how an occupational therapist can influence, support, and change opinions on providing inclusive education in the case study presented in Box 1.1.

BOX 1.1   CASE STUDY: OCCUPATIONAL THERAPIST SUPPORTING INCLUSIVE EDUCATION

An occupational therapist was new to a school district and was assigned to lower elementary grades. She initially began working under a more traditional model of providing "pull-out" services to the students assigned to her caseload. As the year continued, her caseload grew, and it became apparent that in some classrooms more than half the students received occupational therapy services. The occupational therapist spoke with the classroom teacher about coming to the classroom once a week to run an occupational therapy group focused on sensory processing and integration. The teacher agreed that this would benefit all students and a 30-minute time slot was assigned each week as occupational therapy group time.

The occupational therapist was mindful of the students in the classroom who were on her caseload and developed group plans with individual components to address the unique goals of each of the students. She worked closely with the classroom assistant to provide suggestions on how to support those unique goals during the group time while also providing individualized support to the students on her caseload. The teacher was always present during group time, but often was only there to provide support if needed. She was able to use this time to work on other responsibilities, such as documentation and lesson planning. As a result, the teacher saw an immediate benefit to her workload. The occupational therapist was seen as a support to her rather than a burden or extra work.

As the occupational therapist continued to come into the classroom weekly, the teacher was able to see what kinds of activities the occupational therapist chose to perform with the students, and how the occupational therapist modified activities to meet the needs and individual goals of the students on her caseload. The teacher saw improvements in all the students' skills in behavior and academics.

The primary teacher then began to initiate one-on-one meetings with the occupational therapist. These started as informal meetings in the hallway or small discussions after the group time, but these meetings moved to more formal times during the teacher's planning period. The teacher actively sought out the opinions and input of the occupational therapist about many students, including those on the therapist's caseload and other students in the class. Since the occupational therapist was in the classroom, she had already observed all of the students and was familiar with the classroom routines. She could then make skilled recommendations based on the unique needs of students and identify students through universal screening who may be at risk for falling behind and would warrant additional support. The occupational therapist was responsible for documentation and progress monitoring for the group time for students on her caseload. Still, the teacher could also document progress for all students in their other goal areas.

The classroom teacher began talking to other teachers and administrators about how successful this model was for her students and how it eased her workload. As a result, other teachers invited the occupational therapist into their classroom for a designated time each week. Since the occupational therapist tailored the group activities to be specialized towards the goals of the students' IEPs, she was able to consider minutes spent in the classroom as part of the minutes in the IEP. This helped ease her workload, allowed students to stay in the classroom more, supported all students, and facilitated collaboration between the occupational therapist and the teachers. By the end of the school year, nearly all of the teachers had invited the occupational therapist into the classroom to run an occupational therapy group regularly.

The teachers experienced so many benefits of the activities provided in the classroom that they began to ask for more support from the occupational therapist. While her time was limited, the support the teachers were asking for was in the areas of sensory processing and implementation of individualized sensory supports. The teachers and occupational therapist advocated for an additional part-time classroom assistant who would work directly with the occupational therapist. The occupational therapist outlined sensory activities to provide to students and trained this classroom assistant in how and when to administer these activities. She also provided training to the assistant on how to gather data on the activities and identify targeted behaviors. The classroom assistant met with the occupational therapist every day for a few minutes at the beginning and end of the day. The classroom assistant collected data on activities performed and how the students responded. During meetings with the classroom assistant, the occupational therapist reviewed this data to make changes to sensory activities as needed. This model allowed students to receive crucial interventions but did not require direct skilled professionals to implement them. This saved the school district money compared to hiring additional skilled therapy staff while still meeting the needs of the students.

Summary

Before the mid-1970s, many children with disabilities were excluded from public education. Starting in 1975, all children were guaranteed access to public education, thus opening the door for occupational therapy in the school setting. Today, occupational therapy services in the school setting are diverse and are guided by many laws and regulations, and all occupational therapy practitioners must be familiar with these laws as well as state and district guidelines. Occupational therapy is a necessary part of moving toward an inclusive education approach. It plays a vital role in training, collaborating, and modifying the environment to ensure education is inclusive and accessible to all children. The remainder of this book will focus on how the occupational therapy practitioner can support inclusive education when supporting students' sensory needs in the educational setting. We will start by looking at how sensory integration and processing impacts education in the next chapter.

References

American Institutes for Research (AIR) (2024). *Multi-level prevention system.* Center on Multi-Tiered System of Supports. https://mtss4success.org/essential-components/multi-level-prevention-system.

American Occupational Therapy Association (AOTA) (2012). *AOTA practice advisory on occupational therapy in Response to Intervention.* https://www.aota.org/practice/practice-settings/-/media/e7371c748756467ba101d6966bb98eb2.ashx.

American Occupational Therapy Association (AOTA) (2017). Guidelines for occupational therapy services in early intervention and schools. *American Journal of Occupational Therapy, 71*(S2), 7112410010p1–7112410010p1. https://doi.org/10.5014/ajot.2017.716S01.

American Occupational Therapy Association (AOTA) (2020). Occupational therapy practice framework: Domain and process–Fourth edition. *American Journal of Occupational Therapy, 74*(S2), 1–85. https://doi.org/10.5014/ajot.2020.74S2001.

Baumer, N. & Frueh, J. (2021, November 23). *What is neurodiversity?* Harvard Health Publishing. https://www.health.harvard.edu/blog/what-is-neurodiversity-202111232645.

Cahill, S. (2019). Best practices in multi-tiered systems of support. In G. Frolek Clark, J. E. Rioux, B. E. Chandler (eds), *Best Practices for Occupational Therapy in Schools*, 2nd ed., pp. 3–10. AOTA Press.

CAST (2024). *Universal Design for Learning Guidelines version 3.0.* https://udlguidelines.cast.org.

Coates, K. M. (1985). The education of all handicapped children act since 1975. *Marquette Law Review, 51.* https://scholarship.law.marquette.edu/mulr/vol69/iss1/4.

Every Student Succeeds Act (ESEA), Pub. L. No.114–95, 129 Stat. 1802 (2015).

Family Educational Rights and Privacy Act (FERPA), 20 U.S.C. § 1232g (1974).

Health Insurance Portability and Accountability Act (HIPAA) of 1996, Pub. L. No. 104–191 (1996).

Jimenez, T. C., Graf, V. L., & Rose, E. (2007). Gaining access to general education: The promise of universal design for learning. *Issues in Teacher Education*, *16*(2), 41–54.

Law, M., Cooper, B., Strong, S., Stewart, D., Rigby, P., & Letts, L. (1996). The person-environment-occupation model: A transactive approach to occupational performance. *Canadian Journal of Occupational Therapy*, *63*(1), 9–23. https://doi.org/10.1177/000841749606300103.

Nilholm, C. (2020). Research about inclusive education in 2020: How can we improve our theories in order to change practice? *European Journal of Special Needs Education*, *36*(3), 358–370. https://doi.org/10.1080/08856257.2020.1754547.

No Child Left Behind Act of 2001, 20 U.S.C. § 6319 (2002).

Parham, L. D., Roley, S. S., May-Benson, T. A., Koomar, J., Brett-Green, B., Burke, J. P., Cohn, E. C., Mailloux, Z., Miller, L. J. & Schaaf, R. C. (2011). Development of a fidelity measure for research on the effectiveness of the Ayres Sensory Integration® intervention. *American Journal of Occupational Therapy*, *65*(2), 133–142. https://doi.org/10.5014/ajot.2011.000745.

Patten, K. K., Murthi, K., Onwumere, D. D., Skaletski, E. C., Little, L. M., & Tomchek, S. D. (2024). Occupational therapy practice guidelines for autistic people across the lifespan. *American Journal of Occupational Therapy*, *78*(3), 7803397010. https://doi.org/10.5014/ajot.2024.078301.

Piller, A., Teng, K., Andelin, L., Kocher, E., Wiles, A., Niblock, J., Johnson, L. (2023). An overview of school-based sensory interventions using the multi-tiered system of support. *Sensory Integration and Processing Special Interest Section Quarterly*. https://www.aota.org/publications/sis-quarterly/sensory-integration-processing-sis/sispsis-11-23.

Ralabate, P. K. (2011). Universal design for learning: Meeting the needs of all students. *The ASHA Leader*, *16*(10), 14–17. https://doi.org/10.1044/leader.FTR2.16102011.14.

Rioux, J. E. & Chandler, B. E. (2019). History of occupational therapy in schools. In G. Frolek, D. H. Rose, A. Meyer, & C. Hitchcock (eds), *The Universally Designed Classroom: Accessible Curriculum and Digital Technologies*, 2nd ed. Harvard Education Press.

Rose D. (200) Universal design for learning. *Journal of Special Education Technology*, 15(4), 47–51. doi: 10.1177/016264340001500407 .

Schneider, E. & Chandler, B. E. (2019). Laws that affect occupational therapy in schools. In G. Frolek Clark, J. E. Rioux, & B. E. Chandler (eds), *Best Practices for Occupational Therapy in Schools*, 2nd ed., pp. 19–26. AOTA Press.

Section 504, Rehabilitation Act, 29 U. S. C. § 794 (1973).

U.S. Department of Education (2024, February 16). *A history of individuals with disability act*. IDEA: Individuals with Disabilities Education Act. https://sites.ed.gov/idea/IDEA-History.

U.S. Department of Education (2020). *A transition guide to postsecondary education and employment for students and youth with disabilities*. https://sites.ed.gov/idea/files/postsecondary-transition-guide-august-2020.pdf.

U.S. Department of Education (2019, November 7). *Individualized family service plan*. IDEA: Individuals with Disabilities Education Act. https://sites.ed.gov/idea/statute-chapter-33/subchapter-iii/1436.

U.S. Department of Education (2017a, May 2). *Section 300.34 related services*. IDEA: Individuals with Disabilities Education Act. https://sites.ed.gov/idea/regs/b/a/300.34.

U.S. Department of Education (2017b, May 3). *Section 300.111: Child find.* IDEA: Individuals with Disabilities Education Act. https://sites.ed.gov/idea/regs/b/b/300 .111.

Walker, V. L., Conradi, L. A., Strickland-Cohen, M. K., & Johnson, H. N. (2023). School-wide positive behavioral interventions and supports and students with extensive support needs: A scoping review. *International Journal of Developmental Disabilities*, *69*(1), 13–28. https://doi.org/10.1080/20473869.2022.2116232.

Wray, E., Sharma, U., & Subban, P. (2022). Factors influencing teacher self-efficacy for inclusive education: A systematic literature review. *Teaching and Teacher Education*, *117*, 103800. https://doi.org/10.1016/j.tate.2022.103800.

Chapter 2

Sensory Processing and Its Impact on Education

Sensory Integration and Processing

As discussed in Chapter 1, a crucial part of an occupational therapist's role when working in a school setting is to assess, evaluate, support, and suggest unique adaptations for students with different access needs. In order to help teachers and other school personnel provide inclusive education for all, it is important that practitioners understand how sensory processing can impact a student's education, enabling them to offer tailored and targeted recommendations that encourage the student's learning and progress. This chapter will provide an overview of sensory integration and processing, beginning with our eight sensory systems, detailing how they can impact a student's learning and school performance. It will then review the sensory environment, exploring why it is essential that the learning space is an adequate fit and that there is a balance between the person's sensory processing patterns and the sensory features of the environment. Finally, the chapter will discuss sensory integration, examining common sensory strategies that are advantageous in a school setting in comparison to other traditional sensory integration techniques.

What is Sensory Integration and Processing?

A. Jean Ayres, the founder of sensory integration theory, defined sensory integration as "The process by which people register, modulate, and discriminate sensations received through the sensory systems to produce purposeful, adaptive behaviors in response to their environment (Ayres, 1979, as cited in American Occupational Therapy Association [AOTA], 2008, p.1). What this definition tells us is that two separate people may experience the same event, but their bodies may respond and interpret the event differently. Ultimately, they will react in their own unique way based on their sensory processing.

Incredibly, our body and brain are bombarded with sensory stimuli through our many receptors, such as our ears, eyes, and skin, constantly throughout the

DOI: 10.4324/9781032654768-3

day. The sensory receptors take in information about the sensory environment, send this information to the brain, and then support our brain as it processes the information. The brain begins by registering and interpreting the sensory stimuli in the brain's lower regions before moving up to the brain's cortical areas to organize and formulate a response, and then initiates our unique reaction based upon the demands of the environment.

Each child has a unique method of processing sensory information. Let us take the sense of hearing for an example. For one student, they will hear the bell through their receptors (ears), and this information will be registered by their brain. Since the student has assigned meaning to the bell from past experience, they will process that the noise is signaling the start of the school day. This student responds adaptively by going to their desk to sit with their materials. However, another child may hear the bell and have a different response. When the auditory information sends the signal to the brain, the brain interprets this information as noxious or dangerous. Rather than responding adaptively, this may cause the child to react in a fight, flight, or freeze response, such as running away, shouting loudly, or becoming paralyzed with fear.

Often children with sensory processing dysfunction do not have a poor response to sensory stimuli, but rather they have difficulties with processing sensory information. The response is appropriate to how the child processes the information. It is how the brain is processing the sensory information that may be the issue. In the case of the child who responded to the bell in a protective manner (fight, flight, or freeze), the brain interpreted the auditory information as threatening and responded correctly to a dangerous situation. Therefore, the issue was in how the brain processed the sensory input, not in the response. In order to understand this further and see how we can best support students with sensory processing difficulties, it is necessary to understand our eight sensory systems.

Overview of Sensory Systems

There are eight recognized sensory systems within us that help us interact and respond to our environments. Our sensory systems are protective in nature, meaning that they help us interpret how different sensory information will impact our future and attempt to ensure our survival. Our sensory systems also are the driving force behind our engagement with our environment. Some sensory systems are designed to provide information about what happens directly to the person's body (for example, tactile, proprioceptive), whereas other systems are designed to provide information about the environment from a distance (for example, auditory). We will now look at these in turn, starting with the systems responsible for body awareness.

SYSTEMS RESPONSIBLE FOR BODY AWARENESS

The **vestibular system** is considered the movement system of the body, and the receptors are located in the inner ears. Although the receptors are a very small sensory organ, (a bony labyrinth comprised of the vestibule [saccule and utricle] and semi-circular canals), the vestibular system is very important and impactful to a person's sense of self, their spatial awareness and positioning, and their relational understanding of themselves to other aspects of their environment. The vestibular system responds to the pull of gravity and is responsible for providing information on the position of the head, balance, equilibrium, projected actions, and coordinating head and body movements. In addition, the vestibular system directly impacts physiological arousal levels and attention. This is an important consideration, as all humans from birth through older adulthood use movement to change their level of arousal. For example, a baby is rocked to calm them when upset, decreasing their level of arousal. Likewise, an adult may take a walk when almost falling asleep at their desk to increase their level of arousal to finish the workday.

The **proprioceptive system** provides information on body awareness, including the location of the body, the limbs, and how and where the body is moving. The receptors for proprioception are located in the muscles and joints. **The proprioceptive system, with the tactile system, is known as the somatosensory system**. The somatosensory system provides information on body awareness and creates and maintains a map of the body in the brain. Further, the proprioceptive system is responsible for grading the force of movement and providing information on our body positions and movements without the use of vision.

The vestibular and proprioceptive systems work very closely together when responding to sensory input to maintain and move the body through space. Together, the two systems allow the body to maintain an upright position, maintain balance, maintain postural control, control ocular motor movements, coordinate motor movements, and help perform many more "automatic" motor functions. The two systems are so interconnected that they are often evaluated together in a sensorimotor evaluation. The evaluator may provide information on how the systems are processing individually and together to generate a full picture of vestibular and proprioceptive processing.

The **tactile system** is the third sensory system and was foundational in developing the original sensory integration theory (Ayres, 1979). The receptors for the tactile system are the skin, the body's largest sensory organ. It is the first sensory system we develop and provides the initial bonding between an infant and mother. The tactile system is complex and interprets many different types of input beyond just the tactile features of an object. It also provides information on the localization of touch, pain, and temperature. Since the skin is such a large sensory organ, a lot of information is taken in by the tactile system. As a result, hyperreactivity in this system can be very disruptive to a child.

DISTANCE SENSORY SYSTEMS

The visual and auditory systems, known as distance systems, or exteroception, help to provide information to the brain about sensory stimuli away from the body. They are designed to protect the person from potential dangers in their environment, giving their body time to respond to ensure safety. As these two systems are intended to keep a person safe, they take in a lot of information continuously. As a result, a hyperreactive response in either system can be very distressing to a person and can cause the nervous system to be in a state of high alert for much of the time. It can also cause a child to enter a state of fight, flight, or freeze.

The **visual system** is the most dominant and heavily relied upon sensory system. The receptors are the eyes, and information is processed in the visual cortex. The visual system provides information about the environment, including physical features, spatial features, and social cues. Beyond acuity, ocular motor skills and visual perception should be considered when addressing the visual system. The visual and vestibular systems work very closely together with the vestibular-ocular reflex, but it should be noted that the visual system will dominate over the vestibular system. For example, if a person is experiencing seasickness on a boat, they are told to look at the horizon as the horizon does not move. This is because the dominant sensory system (visual) overrides the lesser system (vestibular), helping the person feel less unwell. On the other hand, a person may feel motion sickness in a visually stimulating environment, such as an IMAX movie, even though their body is not moving.

The **auditory system** is another distance system that provides a sense of space and social participation cues. The receptors are the ears, and consequently the auditory and vestibular systems have a close relationship. This is because both sensory systems share the vestibulocochlear nerve (CN VIII). The brain is designed to alert in response to different types of auditory stimuli, which also activates the postural muscles. The auditory system is very important for social interactions as these require hearing acuity (sharpness), auditory discrimination (ability to distinguish words, sounds, and spoken information from background noise), and auditory perception (understanding the properties of sounds), which helps the person understand their environment.

The **olfactory system**, or smell system, relies on the nose as the receptor. The primary olfactory cortex also includes the amygdala, which is the emotional center of our brain (Herz, 2016). Therefore, scents can produce strong emotions that we may associate with memories, providing information about the self and the environment. While the olfactory system is not significant in original sensory integration theory, it is important to consider the emotions that may come up due to different scents and how this may impact a child's learning or response to their environment. Further, a noxious response to olfactory stimuli can impact the ability to perform within an environment optimally.

OTHER SENSORY SYSTEMS

The **gustatory system**, taste, has its receptors in the mouth (i.e. our taste buds) to recognize five tastes: salt, sweet, bitter, sour, and umami. It informs the brain about what type of nutrition a person may gather from the food source and provides a warning for poisons. Many things can impact the taste of foods, including memories, hunger, or fullness, and other visceral responses. The gustatory system plays a prominent role in feeding and eating (Vincis & Fontanini, 2019).

Interoception is the perception of the internal body and encompasses awareness of the visceral aspects of the body. The nervous system registers, interprets, and responds to the information provided by the interoception receptors of the body. In the Occupational Therapy Practice Framework–Fourth edition (AOTA, 2020), interoception is defined as "Internal detection of changes in one's internal organs through specific sensory receptors (e.g., awareness of hunger, thirst, digestion, state of alertness)" (p. 53). The interoception system provides continuous information on the state of the body to the central nervous system to help maintain a state of homeostasis (Schmitt & Schoen, 2022).

Table 2.1 summarizes the eight sensory systems, which you can use for reference as you continue reading. Armed with this knowledge, we will now explore sensory integration and processing.

Overview of Sensory Integration and Processing

Sensory integration and processing has two main aspects: modulation and reactivity, and sensorimotor. Modulation and reactivity refer to how the brain processes the incoming information. Responses exist on a spectrum and may also be dependent upon the expectations of the environment. In all cases, the brain may respond adaptively, or it may overreact or under react.

Table 2.1 Overview of Sensory Systems

Sensory System	Receptors	Main Responsibilities
Vestibular	Organs of the inner ear	Head position Balance Positions in space
Proprioceptive	Muscles and joints	Body awareness Force of movement
Tactile	Skin	Touch
Auditory	Ears	Hearing
Visual	Eyes	Seeing
Gustatory	Tongue (taste buds)	Tasting
Olfactory	Nose	Smelling
Interoception	Internal organs	Internal body sensations (i.e. hunger, thirst, need to use the bathroom, cold, etc.)

When the brain overreacts, this is often referred to as hyperreactivity. This is where the brain responds to stimuli that should be filtered or ignored, or it has a more significant response than expected to the stimuli in that environment. When the brain under reacts, this is often referred to as hyporeactivity. A person is said to have a hyporeactive response when they do not react to sensory input when it would be expected. Every person has different levels of processing each type of sensory stimuli along the spectrum from hyporeactivity to hyperreactivity, and how a person processes sensory information drives their choices of occupations. For example, a person who is more on the hyporeactive side of processing vestibular input may choose a job that involves a lot of movement rather than a desk job. They may have leisure activities that many would consider "risky," such as sky diving, that provide a lot of vestibular stimulation.

Children who are hyperreactive to sensory input frequently are identified as having sensory processing difficulties due to their behavioral responses to sensory input. For instance, a child who is hyperreactive to tactile input may only wear one or two shirts and refuse to wear any others, or cry when their hands get messy. This can be very disruptive to the child's participation in daily activities and to the overall family routine. Often, these children may avoid tasks or environments where the presence of certain sensory stimuli causes their brain to over respond. In an overresponse, the brain may perceive the stimuli as noxious, determining that it should be avoided for safety. Thus, using cognitive strategies to calm them is only effective to a point. If the brain translates sensory stimuli as harmful, it will do anything it can to get the body away from that stimulus as a form of protection. Simply telling the child who is experiencing an overresponsive reaction to sensory stimulation that it is "not too much" or that it will "be okay" does not help calm their nervous system.

Sensory defensiveness is the extreme form of hyperreactivity, such that the brain causes an autonomic nervous system (ANS) response of fight, flight, or freeze. This can be very debilitating to a child and cause avoidance of sensory stimulation, environments, or situations that may involve that type of sensory stimuli. Sensory memories are stored in the brain as a protective response, which can lead to the child over responding to the same stimuli in the future as a defense mechanism. Even after the child works through some sensory processing difficulties, they may continue to avoid situations because the brain is protecting the body based on a "sensory memory" of a past experience.

Below are a few examples of what sensory memory and sensory experience avoidance could look like.

- Not participating in boat-related activities after experiencing seasickness on a childhood holiday.
- Refusing to wear collared shirts if they were uncomfortable in childhood.
- Avoiding carnivals or noisy venues after being startled by a loud noise at a fairground as a child.

On the other hand, children who are hyporeactive need a lot of sensory input in order for their brains to function, process, and respond to sensory stimuli. For example, a child who is hyporeactive to vestibular input may have difficulty sitting still, or refuse to come in from the playground because they want to keep swinging, climbing, and running. It is important to remember that the need for sensory input is an innate need, like food or water. If a child's brain is telling them they need sensory input, then that need must be fulfilled in order for the child to function at the optimal level. This is comparable to when a person is hungry – they may still be able to perform daily activities, but they are not at their optimal performance level. Eventually, the need to eat takes over, and all the person can think of doing is eating. When a child requires sensory input, they also need to satisfy this hunger.

Impact of Sensory Processing on Alertness Levels

As mentioned previously, sensory input impacts a person's alertness level and physiological level of arousal, with different types of input tending to either alert or calm a person. Occupational therapy practitioners design sensory programs to help change a child's level of alertness to match the demands of the task and thus increase their participation. While there are general principles of sensory input, every child is different. Therefore, it is important that each child is individually evaluated by an occupational therapist to ensure the best input is provided to the child when needed. Table 2.2 outlines these general principles of sensory input, showing how different inputs most typically affect the physiological state of arousal of a child.

Sensorimotor Challenges

Sensorimotor challenges consist of postural difficulties and challenges with praxis. Postural difficulties are typically related to difficulties with vestibular and proprioceptive processing, meaning that the person's muscle co-contraction is impacted while maintaining positions against gravity. Children with postural difficulties often have concerns with anti-gravity postural control, balance, poor equilibrium reactions, and coordination difficulties.

Challenges with praxis can also be very debilitating to a child and impact more than just motor performance. In sensory integration, praxis is defined as "the neurological process by which cognition directs motor action (Ayres, 1985, p. 71)." Praxis is a result of the person's unique sensory processing, and it involves the planning, initiation, executing, and terminating of a movement. For all of us, if we decide to move in a particular way the brain takes in sensory information from the environment and formulates a motor response. However, if a person has difficulties in processing vestibular and somatosensory input, the brain may get incorrect information about the environment and the body within

Table 2.2 General Principles of Sensory Input

Sensory System	Type of Input	General Impact on Arousal Level
Vestibular	Linear Rocking Two-point linear swinging	Calming
Vestibular	Vertical (i.e. bouncing, jumping)	Alerting
Proprioception	Climbing Weight bearing Pushing/pulling	Calming
Proprioception: Oral input	Chewing	Calming
Tactile	Light touch	Alerting
Tactile	Deep pressure (e.g. weighted items, "squishes," massage)	Calming
Visual	Flashing lights Bright lights	Alerting
Visual	Low lighting Darker rooms Repetitive visual stimuli (e.g. bubble timers, lava lamps, hour glasses)	Calming
Auditory	Higher pitches	Alerting
Auditory	White noise Music (60 beats per minute)	Calming
Olfactory	Lavender Rose Jasmine	Calming
Olfactory	Peppermint Cinnamon Citrus	Alerting
Gustatory	Sour Spicy	Alerting

the environment. As a result, their response is also inaccurate. With neurological adaptation, the brain may recognize that the motor response will not be successful and modify the motor plan. However, children with sensory-based praxis difficulties may not have another motor plan to utilize. So, although they know the motor plan will be unsuccessful, their brain does not produce an alternative, making them fail at completing the task. Some children do not get the correct information during the execution of the motor plan and also do not recognize the motor plan will be unsuccessful until the task is completed unsuccessfully. For example, a child who trips over a curb may not recognize that they did not pick their foot up high enough over the curb until they hit the ground.

If children struggle with praxis, everyday tasks can be hard for them to complete independently. Children often learn that tasks are hard to complete, but the innate desire for mastery still exists. This can cause children to react in different ways to difficult tasks or tasks they perceive as being problematic. A child with difficulties with praxis may face unsuccessful experiences several times throughout the day, causing them to become easily upset and frustrated. Another child may engage in behaviors that protect them from completing a task where they know they will not succeed. These behaviors may look maladaptive or avoiding, and a child may be labeled a "behavioral problem." Some children become the "class clown," purposefully engaging in activities that are off task, but which provide a positive response from peers through generating laughter. Other children may engage in behaviors that cause them to avoid a situation such as eloping or laying their head on the desk refusing to participate.

With this in mind, it is important to assess praxis and see if this is an area that may be causing a child to have difficult behaviors or not participate in classroom learning. From this, it is evident that sensory processing challenges can have serious impacts on a child's ability to learn.

Sensory and Learning

Sensory processing is the foundation for learning and behavior needed to participate in school. Children take in the information needed for learning through their sensory systems, especially auditory and visual, and rely on sensory processing to maintain attention, positions in space, and a sense of self to make cognitive information meaningful. Children with a poor understanding of their bodies in relation to the world around them may experience anxiety or distress with everyday tasks. Moreover, disruptions in sensory processing may cause children to seek out external control through rigidity in routines or the need for control in situations (Purpura et al., 2022). In other words, if a child does not feel like they have internal control over their bodies, they may seek external control in their environment.

Each person has a finite amount of energy that is able to be used for each task. Some tasks may require more cognitive energy, such as in an academic setting. Others may require more social-emotional energy, such as when engaging in social situations. Play tasks may require more sensorimotor energy (Schkade & Schultz, 1992). If sensory processing dominates a child's finite energy system, there is little energy left for tasks requiring social-emotional or cognitive energy, such as learning and socializing.

If sensory processing overwhelms the finite energy system, a child will seek to regulate using cognitive energy. However, this is only effective to a point. Many children are known to "hold it together" while at school, only to "fall apart" at home. This is an example of using cognition to override sensory processing needs. Still, eventually, it becomes too much for the cognitive system to bear, and the sensorimotor needs overwhelm the child. For example, a child may be hyperactive to vestibular input and need to move. Yet, the child knows they must stay in their seat at school to avoid getting into trouble. They tell their brain to be still and wait, which is effective for a time. However, at some point, the sensory system will take over if the need for movement is unmet.

Children who experience hyperreactivity to sensory input can often be in a state of high alert or stress much of the time. This can cause them to need to focus more cognitive energy on calming and filtering sensory information, thus taxing their cognitive system, which should be used for higher-level learning. It is similar for children with sensory-based motor challenges. If a child struggles with a praxis they use higher levels of their brain to plan and adjust their movements. When children have to use cognitive energy to think about movements that should be automatic, they have less cognitive capacity to focus on learning and social participation. Often, children's sensory processing differences may not appear to be directly impacting their ability to participate in educational activities. However, when the occupational therapist takes a closer look at the whole picture, they may learn that a child is focusing energy on regulation and motor planning, which takes synergy away from the cognition that should be devoted to learning. This is where sensory integration therapy and school-specific sensory-based interventions and strategies can help students.

Box 2.1 describes a sample case of a learner, named Anthony, who demonstrates difficulties in sensory processing and explores how those difficulties may impact his participation in school.

BOX 2.1   CASE DESCRIPTION OF CHILD WITH SENSORY PROCESSING DIFFERENCES AND IMPACT ON EDUCATION

Anthony is seven years old and in the first grade. Overall, he did well in kindergarten, besides some difficulties with behaviors around following directions. However, the teacher thought this was more related to emotional maturity and expected he would catch up with his peers with time. Academically, he had difficulties with letter recognition and writing. His kindergarten teacher suggested some supplemental learning camps during the summer to help fill in the gaps Anthony had exhibited during kindergarten and help him prepare for first grade. Anthony participated in the summer camps but needed help paying attention and staying with the group. The camp leader reported that Anthony had tended to escape from the group to go to the play area or bathroom when that was unexpected. He continued to display difficulties with letter recognition and producing written letters.

When Anthony entered first grade, he had even greater difficulty than he did in kindergarten. He was not keeping up with the assignments, frequently left his desk and wandered around the classroom, often lagged behind when the class was transitioning, and continued to be behind grade level for reading and writing skills. The teacher discussed these concerns with Anthony's parents, and they decided to seek an outside occupational therapy evaluation to examine sensory processing.

Overview of Anthony's Sensory Processing

- **Vestibular**: Anthony demonstrated decreased registration of vestibular input, as evidenced by absent post-rotary nystagmus (PRN), immature equilibrium reactions, and poor balance without the use of his vision.
- **Proprioception**: Anthony has some difficulties with proprioceptive processing, which impacts his ability to grade the force of his movements.
- **Vestibular/proprioception**: Difficulties processing vestibular and proprioceptive input impact Anthony's balance reactions, postural control, ocular motor skills, and sequencing and coordination.
- **Tactile**: He has decreased tactile discrimination, which is required to gain adequate feedback from his environment to generate motor plans efficiently.
- **Auditory**: He also has reported being sensitive to auditory input. Hyperreactivity to sensory input can cause the nervous system to be in a state of high alert, causing a child to spend more cognitive energy on calming and organizing rather than reserving cognitive energy for higher-level learning tasks.
- **Visual**: Anthony has decreased ocular motor skills, which may impact his ability to stabilize his visual field and perform tasks that involve eye movements, such as reading or copying from the board.
- **Motor planning**: Difficulties with sensory processing affect Anthony's motor planning and sequencing. He is not efficiently utilizing incoming sensory input to make adjustments to perform accurate motor movements. As a result, Anthony may need additional time to learn new tasks or additional support to complete tasks. When a task is difficult for Anthony, he may stop the task or try to avoid the task due to difficulties with motor planning.

Summary of Impact of Sensory Processing on Education

Anthony's difficulties with sensory processing impact the following areas of participation in the school setting.

- Maintaining seated and upright positions during desk work.
- Maintaining attention to tasks and regulate arousal level throughout the day.
- Filtering extraneous auditory input to focus on the teacher's instructions.
- Reading and writing skills.
- Following routines of the classroom.
- Performing motor tasks required of first grade students (i.e. writing, cutting, managing his tray in the cafeteria, gathering materials, etc).

Sensory Integration Therapy

Sensory integration therapy is designed to help the brain process sensory information in a more adaptive manner. Ayres Sensory Integration® (ASI), based upon the origination work of A. Jean Ayres is focused on three main principles (Bundy & Lane, 2020).

1) The integration of incoming sensory information is essential for planning and organizing behavior.
2) Difficulties with sensory processing may impede a child's ability to produce appropriate actions, which impacts learning and behavior.
3) The "just right" challenge in integrating sensory information can improve central nervous system (CNS) processing and improve learning and behavior.

ASI is designed to provide enhanced sensory opportunities in the context of child-led play to facilitate an adaptive response. The adaptive response leads to changes in the CNS processing to improve the integration of sensory information. ASI has specific requirements for training and equipment as well as key ingredients essential for the intervention. In Table 2.3, you can see the key components of the ASI fidelity measure (Parham et al., 2011) that distinguish ASI from other interventions that utilize sensory techniques and sensory strategies.

It is important to remember that the goal of ASI is to improve sensory processing. As a result of improved sensory processing, ASI assumes that occupational performance and participation will improve. This frequently differs from the goals of the occupational therapist in the school setting. Here, the occupational therapist is responsible for helping a child access and participate in school activities and daily routines. Therefore, ASI is frequently separate from the interventions provided in the traditional school environment.

Rather, occupational therapists utilize sensory-based interventions and sensory strategies to help a child regulate and organize to complete their school

Table 2.3 Key Ingredients for Ayres Sensory Integration® according to Parham and colleagues (2011).

Key Component	Brief Description
Qualified therapist	Advanced training (post-professional) in sensory integration with at least 50 educational hours; supervision by an advanced practitioner (at least five years experience in sensory integration practice) of at least one hour per month
Comprehensive occupational therapy evaluation	In addition to the required component of occupational therapy, evaluation also includes assessment of the following: • Sensory modulation and discrimination • Postural ocular control • Visual perception and fine motor skills • Motor coordination • Praxis • Organization skills • Influence of sensory integration and processing on performance and linking to referring problems
Physical environment	• Adequate space for equipment and client to engage in gross motor tasks • The ability of the environment to be flexible and change quickly (i.e. put the equipment up or take it down easily) • At least one rotational device • No less than three hooks for suspended equipment • Quiet area • At least one set of bungee cords • Mats, cushions, pillows, etc. • Equipment is adjustable and safe • A variety of sensory equipment is available
Communication with caregivers	Goals are developed in collaboration with the client and caregivers/teachers Caregiver/teacher education is ongoing
Ingredients of sensory integration interventions	1 Ensure the client's physical safety 2 Present multiple sensory opportunities with at least three types of sensory input 3 Help the client attain and maintain the desired level of alertness for the task 4 Present challenges to postural, ocular, oral, or bilateral motor control 5 Present challenges to praxis and organization of behavior 6 Collaborate with the client in activity choices 7 Modify activities to present the just right challenge 8 Ensure activities are successful 9 Support the internal drive of the child to play (be playful) 10 Establish and maintain a therapeutic alliance with the client

day. Sensory-based interventions are defined as "adult-directed modalities that are often applied to the child to improve behaviors associated with modulation disorders" (Case-Smith et al., 2015, p. 135). Although school-based occupational therapists tend to use sensory-based interventions more frequently to help students with modulation difficulties it does not mean that ASI cannot or should not be done in the school setting. ASI has been shown to be effective in improving a child's ability to participate in educational activities. A study by Whiting and colleagues (2023), demonstrated that ASI performed in the school setting with consultation with teachers had significant improvements in the children's functional regulation and active participation. However, it is important that school-based occupational therapy practitioners using ASI in the school system maintain good fidelity to the intervention as outlined by Parham and colleagues (2011).

Sensory-Based Interventions

Table 2.4 presents examples of sensory techniques, including sensory-based interventions and sensory environmental modifications, which school-based occupational therapists can use in their practice. Linking to each of the eight sensory systems, these adjustments can be made available to all students to help them gain the right amount of sensory input they need to succeed in the classroom. In the next section, we will dive deeper into some of these examples and the importance of the sensory environment on students' learning.

Sensory Environment

The sensory environment is crucial to participation in the school setting. For students, the learning space can make or break their ability to engage in their lessons. Therefore, it is important for an occupational therapist to examine and consider the fit between the person and the environment to encourage learning for all.

Every child has different sensory needs and ways of processing sensory input. Modifying the environment creates an opportunity to decrease the need to filter and process extraneous sensory input, which in turn can effectively and positively increase participation. However, it is also important to remember that, since everyone's sensory processing is different, it is impossible to create a sensory environment conducive to all sensory needs. As discussed in Chapter 1, when supporting universal design for learning, having options and different spaces can help provide opportunities for as many different sensory processing patterns as possible. Creating different areas of the classroom that are conducive to sensory needs can be a way to ensure all students have access to their most ideal environment.

Table 2.4 School-Based Sensory Techniques

Sensory System	Sensory-Based Intervention/Environmental Modification
Visual	Light covers
	Lamps instead of overhead lights
	Natural lighting
	Closing the shades
	Dimming lights or turning lights off
	Bubble lamps
	Wearing sunglasses
	Wearing hats to block overhead lights
	Sensory calm-down jars
	Decrease items on walls and desks
	Darker areas of the room, such as a tent
	Color code schedules
	Visual schedules and timers
	Access to visual tools (kaleidoscopes, spinning toys, bubble timers, etc.)
Auditory	Headphones
	Ear plugs
	Cloth headbands over ears or wearing a hood
	Listening to music in headphones
	Calming music (classical or 60 beats per minute)
	Metronomes
	Quiet corner
Tactile	Variety of weighted items (lap pads, blankets, neck weights, ankle weights, etc.)
	Velcro under the desk for students to finger
	Variety of fidgets
	Sensory tables/tubs with various media (i.e. beans, rice, shaving cream, slime, etc.)
	Defined areas for sitting and standing in line to prevent unexpected touch, such as taped squares on the floor or mats for sitting on
Olfactory	A scent-free area in the classroom
	Open windows
	Smelling station with various scented oils
	Calming scents such as lavender using diffusers or candles
Vestibular	Flexible seating options (i.e. rocking chairs, T-stools, balls, move-n-sit cushions, etc.)
	Opportunities to stand at a desk instead of sitting
	Jump and touch station – place a circle on one spot on the wall and allow students to jump and touch that circle
	Head shakes – shake the head back and forth and up and down for quick movement while seated
	Allow for free movement in the classroom

(Continued)

Table 2.4 Continued

Sensory System	Sensory-Based Intervention/Environmental Modification
Proprioceptive	Tie resistance bands to chair legs so students can push their feet on it Chair push-ups Kinesthetic learning opportunities Oral input (chewies, straws, resistive water bottles, etc.) Classroom cleaning activities (putting books away, cleaning the board, cleaning desks, etc.)

One of the most important aspects of creating sensory environments that are conducive to learning is training educators on the impact of the sensory environment. When teachers understand the importance of sensory processing and the sensory environment, they can help design a learning environment that is sensory-friendly and still reflects their values and philosophy of education. It is also important to help teachers understand the importance of seeking feedback from students on the environment and how it impacts their learning. Seeking student feedback is an excellent way to foster neurodiversity-affirming education and ensure student needs are met. Feedback can be gathered formally or informally by simply questioning students while using spaces or providing feedback tools through surveys or questionnaires. In addition, more formal progress monitoring methods designed to examine specific goals can also be used to evaluate the effectiveness of a modified sensory environment as an intervention.

When creating sensory spaces, the spaces should be flexible and adaptable so that students can modify the environment themselves to meet their needs. Sensory needs can vary throughout the day and can change daily, so opportunities for students to easily adjust the environment can improve success in the classroom. Having sensory tools available, such as flexible seating, headphones, fidgets, etc., can give students choice and control. This promotes universal design for learning and autonomy in a student's sensory needs. Additionally, moveable furniture is one way to create different quiet spaces quickly and easily. For example, various seating options that can be moved to other areas of the classroom can allow students to access a seating option as frequently as they need to during the day.

The sensory environment can be modified in many ways to address sensory systems. However, visual and auditory are two of the most important considerations when designing a sensory learning environment. When considering the visual environment, lighting must be assessed and examined. Lighting should be able to be adjusted for brightness, such as using dimmable lights, natural lighting with adjustable shades, and light covers, and glare should be able to be reduced. In addition, the use of different colors, hues, and brightness of bulbs can be an easy way to create different lighting in the room.

Beyond lighting, occupational therapists can recommend other visual modifications to reduce the visual input a child needs to filter. For example, they can use high-contrast colors for text and background on worksheets, walls, and presentation displays, making text and pictures easier to see. When providing visual information, it is advisable to use clear, readable fonts and to provide material in multiple formats, including large print and digital texts. It is also important to minimize clutter on walls and on desks, and the amount of furniture in the classroom should be considered.

The classroom can be a very auditorily stimulating place. To modify the auditory sensory environment, teachers can place sound-absorbing materials such as carpet, curtains, and acoustic panels around the classroom to decrease noise and echoes. They can also provide quiet areas that are accessible at all times for students who need decreased auditory stimuli. The use of assistive listening devices can aid those with hearing impairments and help students who have difficulties with auditory discrimination. The use of captions, transcripts, and supplemental visual materials can help all students access auditory content.

While the visual and auditory environment may be the most important area to consider when designing a classroom for students with different sensory needs, teachers should also consider other sensory systems. For vestibular considerations in a sensory environment, offering flexible seating is a great way to allow students to get increased movement during their day. Seating can be regular desk chairs, standing, balls, t-stools, move and sit discs, rocking chairs, etc. In some circumstances, allowing students the opportunity to move around the classroom as needed is enough for them to get the movement they need to regulate.

Tactile input can be very calming to students, and one way to offer an opportunity for tactile input is to provide sensory buckets with various fidgets and other textured manipulatives for students to use. If the toys are meeting the students' needs, they will use them appropriately and sensibly. Alternatively, teachers can create spaces like "tactile corners" with weighted items, pillows, blankets, etc. so students can take breaks or do quiet activities.

Finally, the consideration of scents in the classroom is important. It may be good to have a scent-free area and a place where calming scents are available. Naturally, the consideration of ventilation is key in all classrooms and provides cleaner, fresher air.

Ultimately, the classroom sensory environment should be flexible and provide multiple opportunities for sensory input. Students should be able to provide feedback on sensory experiences to help the teacher arrange the classroom environment in a way that is most conducive to the students at the time. Teachers should actively seek input from students on their sensory needs and provide various opportunities for students to learn in sensory spaces that meet their needs.

Teacher Training and Coaching

Sensory-based interventions also include teacher and caregiver training on the implementation of sensory-based interventions. A systematic review examined the effectiveness of teacher and caregiver training and coaching methods as an intervention to address sensory processing differences. This review included four studies that demonstrated improvements in caregiver stress, the child's behavior and regulation, and the ability of caregivers to implement interventions with good fidelity (Miller-Kuhaneck & Watling, 2018). More recent research has continued to validate the effectiveness of caregiver-focused training. Sensory interventions coupled with caregiver training produced improved results in quality of life and goal attainment for children with sensory processing differences (Padmanabha et al., 2019; Pashazadeh Azari et al., 2019). Other caregiver-focused training programs considered the Alert Program® for Self-Regulation (Williams & Shellenberger, 1992) and indicated positive results for caregiver knowledge and use of sensory strategies with their children. While there are limited studies that examine the effectiveness of training for teachers, one study did indicate positive results when ASI was paired with teacher consultation (Whiting, Schoen, & Niemeyer, 2023). Occupational therapy practitioners should consider teacher training, coaching, collaboration, and consultation when implementing sensory-based interventions (SBIs). Chapter 7 discusses in detail methods for training and coaching for school personnel in the use of SBIs.

Summary

Humans are sensory beings with various sensory needs that vary throughout the day. Each person's unique sensory processing drives their choices, and their sensory needs must be met to allow for optimal learning and engagement in the classroom. When sensory needs are adequately met, then learning and behavior naturally improve.

There are eight sensory systems to consider: vestibular, proprioception, tactile, visual, auditory, olfactory, gustatory, and interoception. While each person experiences different levels of sensory processing, extremes and differences in sensory processing can impact participation. These are often known as sensory processing challenges and include reactivity/modulation difficulties, sensorimotor difficulties and challenges with praxis. Occupational therapy practitioners are well equipped to address each of these using principles based on sensory integration theory, including ASI, sensory based interventions, and sensory environmental modifications.

Sensory processing impacts learning and school performance, which is why it is integral that occupational therapists and school staff understand and are trained to address these needs. By understanding how different sensory inputs impact a child's sensory processing, school personnel can recognize the importance of creating a sensory environment that helps children participate fully, reducing the amount of energy a child uses to regulate their nervous systems. Instead, they can be in control of their learning environment, improving their academic and behavioral performance in the school setting.

The next chapter will discuss in detail how the occupational therapy practitioner can intervene at various levels of support (population, group, and individual) using the multi-tiered system of supports (MTSS) approach, keeping sensory needs in mind.

References

American Occupational Therapy Association (AOTA) (2008). *Frequently asked questions about Ayres Sensory Integration®.* https://ocde.us/SPED/Documents/OT%20PT%20Continuing%20Education%20Day/AOTA_SI_Fact_Sheet%20.pdf.

American Occupational Therapy Association (AOTA) (2020). Occupational therapy practice framework: Domain and process–Fourth edition. *American Journal of Occupational Therapy, 74*(S2), 1–85. https://doi.org/10.5014/ajot.2020.74S2001.

Ayres, A. J. (1976). *Sensory Integration and the Child.* Los Angeles: Western Psychological Services.

Ayres, A. J. (1985). *Developmental Dyspraxia and Adult Onset Apraxia.* Sensory Integration International.

Bundy, A. C. & Lane, S. J. (2020). Sensory integration: A. Jean Ayres' theory revisited. In A. C. Bundy & S. J. Lane (eds), *Sensory Integration: Theory and Practice,* 3rd ed., pp. 2–20. F. A. Davis.

Case-Smith, J., Weaver, L. L., & Fristad, M. A. (2015). A systematic review of sensory processing interventions for children with autism spectrum disorders. *Autism, 19*(2), 133–148. https://doi.org/10.1177/1362361313517762.

Herz, R. S. (2016). The role of odor-evoked memory in psychological and physiological health. Brain Sci, 19;6(3), 22. doi: 10.3390/brainsci6030022.

Miller-Kuhaneck, H. & Watling, R. (2018). Parental or teacher education and coaching to support function and participation of children and youth with sensory processing and sensory integration challenges: A systematic review. *American Journal of Occupational Therapy, 72,* 7201190030p1–7201190030p11. https://doi.org/10.5014/ajot.2018.029017.

Padmanabha, H., Singhi, P., Sahu, J. K., & Malhi, P. (2019). Home-based sensory interventions in children with autism spectrum disorder: A randomized controlled trial. *The Indian Journal of Pediatrics, 86,* 18–25. https://doi.org/10.1007/s12098-018-2747-4.

Parham, L. D., Smith Roley, S., May-Benson, T. A., Koomer, J., Brett-Green, B. Burke, J. P., Cohn, E. C., Mailloux, Z., Miller, L. J. & Schaaf, R. C. (2011). Development of a fidelity measure for research on the effectiveness of the Ayres Sensory Integration® intervention. *American Journal of Occupational Therapy, 65*(2), 133–142. https://doi:10.5014/ajot.2011.000745

Pashazadeh Azari, Z. P., Hosseini, S. A., Rassafiani, M., Samadi, S. A., Hoseinzadeh, M., & Dunn, W. (2019). Contextual intervention adapted for autism spectrum disorder:

An RCT of a parenting program with parents of children diagnosed with ASD. *Iranian Journal of Child Neurology, 13*(4), 19–35. https://doi.org/10.22037/ijcn.v13i4.21156.

Purpura G, Cerroni F, Carotenuto M, Nacinovich R, Tagliabue L. (2022). Behavioural differences in sensorimotor profiles: A comparison of preschool-aged children with sensory processing disorder and autism spectrum disorders. *Children*, 9(3), 408. https://doi.org/10.3390/children9030408.

Schkade, J. K. & Schultz, S. (1992). Occupational adaptation: Toward a holistic approach for contemporary practice, part 1. *American Journal of Occupational Therapy, 46*(9), 829–837. https://doi.org/10.5014/ajot.46.9.829.

Schmitt, C. M. & Schoen, S. (2022). Interception: A multi-sensory foundation of participation in daily life. *Frontiers, 16.* https://doi.org/10.3389/fnins.2022.875200.

Vincis, R. & Fontanini, A. (2019). Central taste anatomy and physiology. *Handbook of Clinical Neurology, 164*, 187–204. doi: 10.1016/B978-0-444-63855-7.00012-5.

Whiting, C. C., Schoen, S. A., & Niemeyer, L. (2023). A sensory integration intervention in the school setting to support performance and participation: A multiple-baseline study. *American Journal of Occupational Therapy, 77*, 7702205060. https://doi.org /10.5014/ajot.2023.050135.

Williams, M.S. & Shellenberger, S. (1992). An Introduction to "How Does Your Engine Run?"® The Alert Program® for Self-Regulation [Booklet]. TherapyWorks, Inc.

Chapter 3

Multi-Tiered System of Supports and Occupational Therapy and Sensory Needs

Introduction

As discussed in Chapter 1, schools that receive federal funding are now required by law to offer a multi-tiered system of supports (MTSS) in public education, reducing barriers to education and providing layers of assistance for all students. Therefore, it is crucial that occupational therapists working in school-based settings understand what the tier system is, how it can help students with sensory processing needs, and what interventions and assessment methods are available to ensure students are receiving the appropriate support.

This chapter will review the MTSS, exploring interventions at the school/classroom level (Tier 1), the small group level (Tier 2), and the individual level (Tier 3). We will review and describe each tier in turn before examining and defining how occupational therapy services are evaluated and implemented at each tier, specifically focusing on addressing sensory integration and processing needs. Finally, we will discuss what aspects to consider and how when choosing a tier.

Multi-Tiered System of Supports

The MTSS was introduced as part of the Every Student Succeeds Act in 2015, and it expanded previous laws to go beyond the traditional Response to Intervention (RTI) model. Still, it remained focused on ensuring that all children are performing academically at their grade level by providing academic help as well as social and emotional support. RTI still guides the tiered approach, which is where support is firstly provided to all students in a school or class (Tier 1) before moving up to more targeted small group support (Tier 2). This is for students who have been identified as at risk of falling behind or those who require additional support beyond what is offered in the general classroom and curriculum. If a more targeted intervention is needed for identified students, individual support can then be given at Tier 3. The MTSS intervention model starts in Tier 1 at the population level as a proactive and preventative approach. Tier 2 is a

DOI: 10.4324/9781032654768-4

rapid response approach with high-efficiency interventions at the group level. Tier 3 is a more extended, more intensified approach to individualized interventions at the individual level (American Occupational Therapy Association [AOTA], 2012).

Occupational therapy practitioners have a role in each of the tiered levels under MTSS to meet various student needs. As part of the interdisciplinary team, the occupational therapy practitioner interacts with other professionals to support students at all levels. At Tier 1, the occupational therapy practitioner may contribute to staff training on sensory processing, assist in modifying the sensory environment, and help plan school and classroom routines to provide the best sensory routines for the school and classroom. They can work with school administrators and teachers to develop sensory interventions for all students and support staff in understanding when and how to implement these interventions. In addition, occupational therapists can be part of the universal screening process to help identify students who may need more targeted support.

At a Tier 2 level, the occupational therapy practitioner can assist with the identification of students who have additional sensory needs that impact their ability to participate in educational activities. They can help design group-based interventions to focus on providing additional sensory input to support academic and behavioral needs. Also, occupational therapists can be involved in modifying different aspects of the sensory environment within the larger classroom setting to create sensory spaces that may be more conducive to learning for groups of identified students.

At a Tier 3 level, the occupational therapy practitioner provides more individualized and specialized interventions. This is often thought of as a more traditional model of occupational therapy services that are provided on a one-on-one basis to address goals in an individualized education program (IEP). Goals supported by occupational therapy may be addressed only by the occupational therapy practitioner or by the collaborative team. As a related service, occupational therapy may have goals only related to occupational therapy interventions, or it may embed its support within other goals. For example, in one IEP the occupational therapist may write a goal for maintaining upright positions while seated at a desk. In this case, the occupational therapy practitioner would work on postural control, core activation, and attention and focus to sit at a desk during academic tasks. In another IEP, the occupational therapy practitioner may address the same concept of upright seated positions but may not have a specific goal to address this area. Instead, they may work on a note-taking goal in the IEP to support the posture and attention needed to take sufficient notes from both a motor and executive functioning standpoint. Under a Tier 3 intervention model, occupational therapy practitioners would implement more individualized interventions approaches, such as Ayres Sensory Integration®, but sensory-based interventions can and should be implemented at all tier levels.

There are specific requirements for the implementation of supports under MTSS. It is a preventative model, meaning that the goal of MTSS is to support academics and behavior within the school-setting before students fall too far behind. Therefore, universal screenings, which we will explore in detail later, are an essential component of MTSS.

Each tier in MTSS is a different level of intensity for intervention and instruction, which is why progress monitoring is another required component of MTSS. Progress monitoring must be frequent and ongoing. The goal is to assess student performance, provide quantitative data on the response to implemented interventions, and examine the effectiveness of interventions. The information determines whether interventions should be continued, modified, or discontinued. The progress monitoring should be planned in advance, considering how to measure effectiveness, frequency of data collection, and how to ensure the fidelity of data collection.

Finally, data-based decision-making should be present in all phases of MTSS, including screenings, progress monitoring, and decision-making based on data collection. We will consider each of these components of MTSS in more depth later in the chapter, including how to develop evidence-based interventions.

Along with these essential components, the occupational therapy practitioner is a key part of the interprofessional collaboration team for MTSS. This team comprises all school personnel, including teachers, assistants and aids, occupational and physical therapists, and speech-language pathologists. These teams are designed to solve problems with learning and behaviors in the school setting. The team's first goal is to identify problems and generate a hypothesis as to why the problem is occurring and how to improve the child's performance. Problems are often first identified during the universal screening process. Teams then develop and implement a plan of evidence-based interventions. After a certain amount of time, the team reviews the data gathered, which should be systemic and targeted, and evaluates the effectiveness of the plan in solving the problem. They can then decide how to adjust the interventions based on the progress monitoring. Progress monitoring is a systematic and targeted method of gathering data to determine the effectiveness of an intervention across time.

Prevalence of Sensory Processing Differences

Occupational therapy practitioners frequently work with children with sensory processing differences. These children may have many difficulties in the school setting, including problems with attention, sequencing, participation in classroom routines, and completing assignments. Social participation may also be difficult for children with sensory processing differences, and these children may also struggle with behavioral regulation. As explored in Chapter 2, sensory processing challenges is not typically recognized as a single stand-alone disorder but rather a cluster of symptoms that may accompany another diagnosis, such as autism spectrum disorder (Mulligan et al., 2021). However, some children experience sensory processing challenges that do not meet the criteria for other diagnoses. Neuroimaging studies have shown differences in children with sensory processing challenges and no other etiology, suggesting a distinct difference in neurobiology for children with sensory processing challenges even if no other diagnosis is warranted (Borkowska, 2017).

This being said, the estimates on the prevalence of sensory processing challenges vary due to the lack of agreement on diagnostic criteria, and whether or not these challenges exists in isolation or only as a part of another disorder. Current estimates indicate that between 5–25% of children experience sensory processing challenges (Ben-Sasson et al., 2009; Jussila et al., 2020), with a higher incidence in children with developmental disorders (Jussila et al., 2020). Under the MTSS model, Tier 2 interventions are often required for approximately 15% of the population. This aligns with the statistics on the prevalence of children with sensory processing challenges indicating that many students within the general education setting could be in need of sensory interventions.

Each person has unique sensory processing patterns that exist on a spectrum. While a child may not fall into the category of sensory processing disorder, each individual has unique sensory processing that may or may not be conducive to the current sensory processing requirements of the school setting. In fact, it is important to not always view sensory processing differences as a disorder or maladaptive issue. Instead, the unique sensory processing of a child contributes to their choices in occupations and their strengths as an individual. Difficulties can occur only when there becomes a mismatch between the environmental demands and the child's sensory processing (Dean et al., 2022). If the child or the environment can adapt to increase the fit, then there may be no disorder (Law et al., 1996). Under the MTSS model, the general population of students who do not typically need interventions is about 80%. In this 80% of the school population, occupational therapists may see children with different sensory processing patterns. Providing a proactive and preventative sensory program within the school and classroom setting can help ensure all students can experience the best fit between their own sensory processing patterns and the sensory demands of the school environment.

Before we look at each of the tiers in detail, it is important to understand the importance of universal screening in deciding on the necessary support for each student.

Universal Screening

Universal screenings are one of the essential components of MTSS that school districts must provide on a regular basis. Screenings are performed for all students, both from school-wide and in specific classroom perspectives (AOTA, 2012).

They are often conducted three times a year depending on the school district. Their main purpose is the early identification of students who are at risk of falling behind in academic, social, behavior, or emotional areas. However, other purposes include evaluating the effectiveness of current interventions, curriculum, and instruction, providing data on how to utilize resources most effectively, providing data for reporting to key stakeholders, maximizing state assessment performance, and reducing the chance for over referrals for special education evaluations.

Occupational therapists can utilize the universal screening process to examine students' sensory needs and monitor how current school-wide sensory interventions match the students' requirements. This is achieved by screening the students and examining the sensory environment. The main goal at this point in the MTSS process is to identify if sensory supports can be included within the general education setting to further help students with higher sensory needs. Due to the unique perspective of the occupational therapist and specifically their understanding of sensory processing, sensory needs, and the environment, they play an essential role in the universal screening process to help establish school-wide interventions and identify students who may need more targeted interventions. Figure 3.1 provides a screening checklist for occupational therapists to use when examining the need for sensory interventions, but they can also utilize standard school screening forms if the district prefers. Through the screening process, students identified as having potential needs can be further screened by the occupational therapist to see if sensory supports may improve their academic performance.

However, occupational therapists may have limited time to complete these universal screenings due to high caseloads and working with students who need more direct support. One way to address this is to have other staff perform the general screening, including a screening for sensory needs. This information can be brought to the occupational therapist, who can then decide if further screening is warranted to assess sensory-related issues that may impact student performance. This can help the occupational therapist prioritize their time and work with the team to help as many students as possible.

Figure 3.1 is an observation checklist for assessing the sensory environment. It allows the observer to indicate if a feature is present or not in the categories of lighting, sounds, smells, movement, visual, and tactile/proprioceptive. The checklist provides a column for additional comments.

After a universal screening has been completed, whole school populations and individual students can be assigned to different tiers of support depending on their identified needs. We will now look at each tier and their relevant interventions, as well as how these interventions should be aligned with the Occupational therapy practice framework: Domain and process –Fourth edition (OTPF-4) (AOTA, 2020). The OTPF-4 is the guiding document from AOTA

Location: _____

Date/Time of Observation: _____

Sensory Component	Present	Comments
Lighting Adequate lighting Areas with lower lighting Adjustable lighting	y n y n y n	
Sound Quiet areas available Echoes Sound dampening Amplification device available	y n y n y n y n	
Smells Scent-free areas Areas with calming scents	y n y n	
Movement Opportunities for movement Alternative seating Spaces in the classroom to stand or pace	y n y n y n	
Visual Free of clutter Lots of items on the walls	y n y n	
Tactile/Proprioceptive Fidgets available Weighted items available Oral input available Opportunities for heavy work	y n y n y n y n	

Additional Comments:

Observer Name and Signatur: _____

Figure 3.1 Sensory environment checklist.

that defines and outlines the scope of occupational therapy practice. We will use this document to explain MTSS within the context of occupational therapy's scope of practice and through the occupational therapy process.

Multi-Level Prevention System

Tiered Interventions in Alignment with OTPF-4

The OTPF-4 (AOTA, 2020) outlines the occupational therapy process in three aspects: evaluation, intervention, and targeted outcomes. This process should occur regardless of whether the client is a person, group, or population that matches the clients defined in the OTPF-4 at each tier level under MTSS. At the population level, which aligns with Tier 1, occupational therapists provide evaluations and interventions to school or classroom settings. The population of the school or classroom is the client. At the group level, which aligns with Tier 2, the occupational therapist provides evaluations and interventions for small groups of students with similar needs or experiences. Interventions are designed with the group in mind, and outcomes are focused on the group as the client, although the occupational therapist also considers the impact of each individual on the group as a whole. At the person level, which aligns with Tier 3, interventions are provided to an individual person considering their specific needs. The OTPF-4 provides a clear framework of the occupational therapy process for different types of clients in a clearly defined manner. While all types of clients are considered at all times in occupational therapy, by explicitly looking at a population, group, and persons, the OTPF-4 creates a clear framework for MTSS interventions. Table 3.1 provides examples of the domains of occupational therapy as they relate to person, group, and population levels of clients in alignment with MTSS levels.

Performance skills are also an aspect of the domain of occupational therapy. They allow a client to engage with their environment to perform chosen occupations. Performance skills are goal-directed actions that impact the quality and success of participation in occupations. Examples of performance skills that may be important in school-based occupational therapy include motor skills, process skills, and social interaction skills (AOTA, 2020). While performance skills should be considered in all three levels of clients (population, group, and person) the occupational therapist must recognize that performance skills are unique to the individual. When addressing performance skills in a group or population they are considered according to how they impact the group. For example, a child who has difficulties processing proprioceptive input may participate in social interactions with other students but break their toys. This would cause a response from the group, either to change the toys and materials to items that are less likely to break or to only provide the child with proprioceptive processing difficulties soft toys that cannot be easily broken. The group dynamics,

Table 3.1 Application of OTPF-4 to MTSS Levels

	Person / Tier 3	Group / Tier 2	Population / Tier 1
Client	Child receiving occupational therapy services for 30 minutes each week under an IEP	Group of four second grade students who have been identified as having a higher need for movement in order to participate in class activities	Ms. Johnson's second grade class
Occupation Play	Child swinging at recess	Group of students playing tag at recess	School-wide field day
Performance Patterns Routines	Child in Ms. Johnson's class that receives special education services through an individual daily work schedule/routine	Group of students in Ms. Johnson's class who receive extra support through a reading and math daily schedule/routine	Ms. Johnson's daily schedule/routine for her second grade class
Client Factor	Child's sensory profile	Group of students who are hyporeactive to vestibular input	Highly intensified movement at recess causes the students to need calming input after recess before starting academics

Table 3.2 Sensory Interventions by Client Type

Person	Group	Population
Tier 3	Tier 2	Tier 1
Individual support for sensory processing needs through a sensory diet	Providing a sensory group two times a week for a group of students with sensory processing needs	Providing classroom sensory strategies that the teacher implements every day after lunch to help students focus for the afternoon

participation, and performance skills are impacted by one individual member's performance skills. This means that even when evaluating the client as a group or population, the occupational therapist must consider the performance skills of each individual within the group or population.

Table 3.2 provides an example of a sensory intervention provided at each Tier and how it aligns with the clients as defined by the OTPF-4.

TIER 1

Tier 1 interventions are designed to be preventative and proactive. They are intended to support all students' needs, helping to increase academic performance as well as boosting their behavioral and social skills at school. Under Tier 1, interventions are often designed to identify strengths and build upon them using a strength-based approach, such as implementing a school-wide positive behavioral support plan. In education, using a strength-based approach values a student's positive effort and achievements rather than their mistakes (Lopez & Louis, 2009). It functions under a growth mindset (Dweck, 2010), which views the brain as an organ that grows, much like a muscle. Instead of focusing on deficits, a growth mindset encourages us to focus on learning during each opportunity, even those that are difficult or when errors are made. This contrasts with a fixed mindset that views intelligence as a characteristic that cannot be changed (Garwood & Ampuja, 2018). It is important for educators to have a growth mindset and to facilitate that mindset within their students. Providing school-wide strategies from a strength-based perspective can help all students and educators change their mindset from fixed to growth, creating a positive, non-judgmental environment in which students can improve their performance. Sensory interventions that support the general education curriculum and common core standards should build on a child's strengths and help them move toward success in all areas of education (Cahill, 2019).

Tier 1 interventions are performed in school-wide and individual classrooms, which is what we consider the population level. Populations have similar person factors, such as age, but may also have individual differences, although the individuals within the population should only be considered within the context of the population (AOTA, 2020). Under Tier 1, the occupational therapist should view the school or classroom as a whole as the client, which will guide the evaluation and intervention process. This is important to understand because when working with a client that consists of a population, it is appropriate to examine the performance skills at the person level, as that person exists within the population. However, this is done in the context of the population and how the individual factors impact the function of the population. Occupational therapy services performed at the level of the population are considered skilled therapy services and should follow the occupational therapy process, which consists of evaluation, intervention, and outcomes (AOTA, 2020).

Under Tier 1, considerations for both the school population and the classroom population may be considered. As the focus is on prevention, implementing population-based sensory interventions can be very helpful in supporting improved behavior and maximizing learning. Since all individuals have different sensory processing patterns, the occupational therapist must understand sensory processing from a population perspective and examine the environment. To follow the occupational therapy process, occupational therapists must first initiate an evaluation to determine the unique and multifaceted needs of the population. Chapter 4 will provide more in-depth information on the evaluation process, but universal screenings are an important part of Tier 1 for the valuable information they can provide on the sensory needs of students.

Theoretically, the Person-Environment-Occupation (PEO) theory (Law et al., 1996) provides an excellent approach to guide the intervention process under Tier 1. This theory examines the fit between the person and the environment and seeks to increase this fit so that, in turn, occupational performance will improve. With the PEO approach, the first intervention is within the environment, which is deemed the easiest to change. According to the OTPF-4 (AOTA, 2020), environmental factors are comprised of physical, social, and attitudinal aspects that surround the client, which, in this case, is the population of the school or classroom. Under Tier 1, the occupational therapist can provide interventions designed to modify the sensory environment, which is part of the physical factors of the school setting. The occupational therapist can also help adjust the social environment from a sensory perspective based on how students and school personnel interact.

For example, interventions the occupational therapist might perform at this tier include the following.

- Staff training on sensory processing and sensory supports.
- The development of a school-wide sensory program to embed within classroom routines.
- The evaluation of specific environments, such as individual classrooms, cafeterias, and playgrounds to generate suggestions to modify the sensory environment to provide access for all students.
- Providing services for teachers that address how to consider sensory processing in classroom management.

To maintain the skilled aspect and best practice of occupational therapy, occupational therapy practitioners must have a solid understanding of how to implement occupational therapy services at the population level. Evaluation is essential, as this is the first step in the occupational therapy process. It also aligns with the laws governing MTSS interventions by allowing for data-based decision-making. Evaluation guides the intervention process and provides the data the occupational therapist needs to design skilled interventions. The absence of evaluation data promotes blanket sensory strategy suggestions and general sensory environmental modifications that are not tailored to the population's unique needs. Anyone can utilize the internet or read a book on sensory strategies and implement them. Only the occupational therapist has the knowledge, training, and skills to provide a skilled evaluation of the sensory needs of a population and design unique, skilled interventions that address the needs of that targeted population. An attitudinal shift toward how interventions are designed for sensory processing and the sensory environment must take place to ensure that evidence-based interventions are implemented in accordance with best practices. Practical strategies for promoting these attitudinal changes are discussed later in this book.

To summarize, sensory interventions and strategies at the Tier 1 level consist of implementing additional sensory opportunities throughout the day, developing a sensory routine to promote optimal states of alertness of students to match the classroom routines, and modifying the sensory environment to promote an environment for optimal learning and focus. The occupational therapist engages in screenings and evaluations to provide skilled sensory interventions to promote the participation of all students.

TIER 2

Tier 2 is the next level of intervention in MTSS and provides targeted interventions for students identified as needing additional support. Students may need academic, behavioral, or social-emotional support, and are typically identified during the school-wide screening process. There is an assumption that approximately 20% of students would benefit from Tier 2 interventions, with approximately 5% of those students requiring more intensified interventions at the Tier 3 level (AOTA, 2012).

Interventions at this level of support are standardized and evidence-based, and the occupational therapist plays an important role in their design and development. Most notably, if occupational therapy practitioners are allotted the time and resources to train staff, it may not be necessary for the occupational therapy practitioner to implement these interventions directly. Rather, they can design and monitor interventions for Tier 2 levels of support and provide support, training, and direct intervention when needed to ensure the successful implementation of group interventions.

It is crucial at Tier 2 that groups are small, with no more than 3–7 students, and newly introduced Tier 2 interventions should be provided along with the continued Tier 1 interventions. As always, progress monitoring should occur using a structured and concise method, but a new, vital component of Tier 2 is family involvement. By developing methods of communication with parents and caregivers, occupational therapist practitioners can ensure there is carryover of these interventions in the home environment. In addition, families should be kept informed about their child's progress and if current interventions are effective in improving performance in the school setting. Building this communication and trust with the student's caregivers will allow them to have more capacity for understanding when more or less intensive interventions are needed, especially if the child needs to change tiers of support.

Implementing the occupational therapy process at a Tier 2 level aligns with the OTPF-4 process for clients identified as a group. Groups are made up of individuals that impact the group's dynamics and goals, and interactions between members. For example, if a group of students were participating in a game of freeze tag where two group members used a wheelchair, the group would make sure to play on a surface that was easily accessible to those who used a wheelchair and those who did not. The group may also modify the rules of the game depending on the group members. Therefore, according to the OTPF-4, when addressing the performance skills and client factors, such as sensory processing, the occupational therapist must consider both the individual group members and the group as a whole. The occupational therapist will determine the goal of the group and the relationship of the individual group members to the overall participation of the group. Therefore, assessment of the group would include the individual's sensory processing, both strengths and areas of weakness, as well as how each group member's sensory processing contributes to the overall goal of the group (AOTA, 2020). Putting these pieces together, the occupational therapist can develop a sound intervention plan to address the sensory needs of all students. The occupational therapist should regularly examine progress monitoring to evaluate effectiveness, design changes to the program, and implement additional training if needed.

Sensory interventions at a Tier 2 level are more tailored to the group's needs than interventions at the Tier 1 level. As discussed in Chapter 2, the vestibular, proprioceptive, and tactile systems are the cornerstone of the original sensory integration theory, so providing interventions that incorporate these systems can help students with sensory reactivity and sensorimotor difficulties. For example, deep pressure tactile interventions are key to calming, and these can be implemented at a small group level to help students calm down in school settings.

Another method of implementing Tier 2 interventions is to allow students receiving Tier 3 interventions to participate in Tier 2 group interventions. For instance, a student receiving Tier 3 occupational therapy services could design a sensory group activity to complete with students receiving Tier 2 support while supervised by an occupational therapist. This can provide a way for the student receiving individual services under Tier 3 to apply skills learned in therapy, such as executive functioning, social participation, motor planning, and independence in identifying and implementing sensory strategies. It also allows students receiving Tier 2 sensory interventions to receive sensory supports, all under the guidance of the occupational therapy practitioner. Box 3.1 provides an example of a student receiving individual services under Tier 3 leading a group.

BOX 3.1 BLENDING TIER 2 AND TIER 3 SERVICES

Molly was a fifth-grade student with Down's Syndrome who received direct occupational therapy services under her IEP. Her IEP goals related to occupational therapy included goals focused on fine motor skills, motor planning, and sequencing. She enjoyed working with other students and had been participating in yoga exercises as part of her occupational therapy and classroom routine for strength and self-regulation. Her occupational therapist had also been working with a group of five third-grade students on motor planning, self-regulation, and sequencing. Once a week, they participated in small group time with the occupational therapist for approximately 20 minutes. The occupational therapist knew that yoga would benefit the students as it had Molly.

She decided to ask Molly to design and lead this small group yoga once a month. Molly worked with the occupational therapist to design the yoga program to fit within the time frame, and she practiced the social aspect of leading a group and learned new yoga techniques to teach the small group. Once a month, when the group of students receiving Tier 2 supports participated in their small group yoga time, Molly helped the occupational therapist lead the group's yoga routine. The occupational therapist facilitated the students and modified activities to meet their needs as required, while Molly led the group through a series of yoga moves. Molly worked on her individual IEP goals and helped the students who were receiving services at the Tier 2 level, while the occupational therapist directed and facilitated all students in the group.

TIER 3

Tier 3 is typically considered traditional occupational therapy performed in a one-on-one situation, or small groups with interventions designed to address the individualized goals of each student. Services are implemented under an IEP to ensure students receive the services minutes and services outlined in their IEP. While educational in nature, this model reflects a similar services model to that of the medical setting. In fact, many school districts can bill state Medicaid services for services provided under the IEP.

While an essential part of the occupational therapist's role in the school setting, Tier 3 interventions should be reserved for students with more significant or complex needs that cannot be addressed in a population or group setting. Occupational therapy caseloads are high, with more and more students being identified as having needs that can be supported by occupational therapy. By incorporating occupational therapy at Tier 1 and Tier 2, occupational therapy practitioners are better able to allot their time to students who have more complex needs that require individualized interventions. This can reduce caseload size and afford the occupational therapy practitioner the time to provide truly skilled services rather than just fulfilling IEP minutes. While Tier 3 is essential for many students, the aim of this book is to provide an outline of how to implement services at the Tier 1 and Tier 2 levels in order to allow occupational therapy to influence all students, ensuring practitioners have the time to provide skilled, individualized interventions to those who truly need it.

We will now look at how occupational therapists can develop and implement these interventions, specifically addressing sensory processing needs.

Developing Evidence-Based Sensory Interventions

Many sensory interventions can be utilized in the classroom or school environment, and it is the role of the occupational therapy practitioner to suggest and implement evidence-based interventions rather than simply providing general sensory activities. These evidence-based interventions must be based on three main components: the clinical expertise of the occupational therapist, the student's needs and preferences, and the best available published evidence.

The first step in developing evidence-based sensory interventions for the occupational therapist is to identify sensory needs through assessment. There are several assessment methods that can be used, not all of which are formal or targeted at a particular student, and these assessments can work in collaboration with other professionals to assess the environment, routines, and classroom population. These different assessment methods will be explored fully in Chapter 4.

Additionally, occupational therapists should keep up with current research in sensory integration and interventions to inform their evidence-based suggestions. By reading peer-reviewed publications on sensory interventions, such as the *American Journal of Occupational Therapy,* and other resources that provide summations of and updates on evidence, such as the Collaborative for Leadership in Ayres Sensory Integration®[1], they can ensure they are always adhering to best practice. Further, AOTA offers synthesized evidence in the form of clinical practice guidelines to provide practitioners an appraisal of current evidence and how it can be used within practice. While the previous clinical practice guidelines related to sensory integration, including ASI and sensory-based interventions, were published in 2015 (Watling et al., 2018), new clinical sensory practice guidelines from AOTA were made available in 2025 as an open access document on the AOTA website. Alongside this, clinicians should have working knowledge of current practice guidelines for sensory interventions and school-based practice available from national and state organizations.

Armed with the evidence and an evaluation of needs, occupational therapy practitioners are well prepared to develop an intervention plan to address sensory needs, tailoring the intervention plan to each tier level based on their

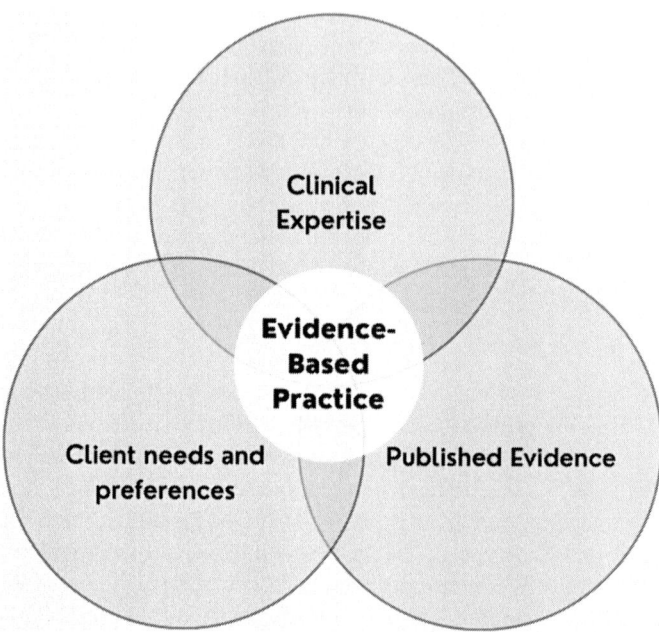

Figure 3.2 Evidence-based practice. Image by author.

client. The occupational therapy practitioner needs to be considerate of the level they are addressing and ensure the intervention applies to the client at that tier, whether it be the population (Tier 1), group (Tier 2), or individual (Tier 3) level. Also, goals should be measurable and focused on empowering clients toward participation, improving functional outcomes, and increasing occupational performance.

An essential element of implementing these evidence-based sensory interventions is training those who are overseeing them, such as teachers and other school personnel. Without proper training on when and how to implement them, interventions will lack fidelity and may not meet the client's needs. In addition to this, appropriate training and follow-up ensures that progress monitoring and relevant documentation is accurate during the assessment, allowing for adjustments to the intervention to be made as needed. By adhering to these three aspects of evidence-based practice, clients can receive the best sensory interventions that meet their needs.

Figure 3.2 is a Venn diagram representing evidence-based practice as the overlap of clinical expertise, client needs and preferences, and published evidence, which allows practitioners to provide the best possible outcomes.

Progress Monitoring

Progress monitoring is a requirement under MTSS, and it allows for decisions to be made regarding the continuation or adjustments needed in interventions. A systematic approach to monitoring progress allows data to be collected and interpreted with confidence. Since the occupational therapy practitioner may not be performing the interventions at a Tier 1 and Tier 2 level, it is even more important to establish a standardized process to ensure quality data.

Progress monitoring should be consistent and ongoing, typically occurring every two to eight weeks (Cahill, 2019). However, data collection may need to happen more frequently. The interprofessional team makes the formal decision on how frequently to monitor progress, and they must ensure there are adequate data points to inform these decisions. Alongside this, district policies may also dictate the frequency of progress monitoring, and data collection may vary in the treatment process. For example, the team may want to gather data on a weekly basis initially to determine if the intervention needs to be modified or continued. Once the determination to continue has been made, the frequency of data collection may decrease to monthly.

Data should be compared to baseline data to determine the effectiveness of the intervention. As student performance fluctuates based on various factors, multiple data collection opportunities must occur before making a decision about effectiveness. Traditionally, at least eight data points should be collected before deciding the effectiveness of the intervention and whether to continue, modify, or terminate the intervention (Cahill, 2019). Providing a systematic process for gathering data for progress monitoring is critical to ensuring that the data is accurate and consistent with intent. A step-by-step process, as outlined below, can help ensure the data is valid (American Institutes for Research [AIR], 2024).

Example: The student will improve on-task behaviors as demonstrated by completing desk work for at least 30 minutes without getting up from their seat.

Step one: Define the behavior that is to be monitored
The behavior to be monitored in this example is how many times a child gets up from their seat during 30 minutes of desk work.

Step two: Define what data will be collected
This defines the measurement strategy, including duration, frequency, intensity, length of time, etc. In the example provided, the measurement strategy is frequency counts. The data collector will tally the number of times the student gets up from the desk during a 30-minute period.

Step Three: Gather baseline data

Baseline data should be collected across settings and at various times during the day. This means that the data collection should occur in any environment where the student is required to perform seated desk work and at various times during the day, such as morning, after lunch, and afternoon. If possible, the same data collection person should be used across times and settings to ensure valid data collection. Enough data should be collected to ensure a valid baseline has been established.

Step four: Implement the intervention

This step includes additional assessment, development of the intervention, and training staff on how and when to implement the intervention.

Step five: Establish the timeline for data collection

Have a written plan for when data collection should occur and who is responsible for ensuring data collection.

Step six: Train staff on the data collection procedure

Provide training on the data collection method and a timeline for when data collection should occur.

Step seven: Plot the data

Remember, performance fluctuates, so it is important to have many data points. The best approach is to plot these data points in a graph so that trends are more visible, as seen in Figure 3.3.

Figure 3.3 provides a visual representation of a sample progress monitoring chart to track goals using generic sample goals over an eight-week period. The chart provides a line graph of three goals showing a fluctuation for goal 1, gradual improvements for goal 2, and highest starting values with variance over time for goal 3. This chart is useful for tracking and visualizing progress in measurable goals.

Step eight: Analyze the data

Examine data plots using an interprofessional approach and discuss trends. Match data points with aspects of the environment, including time of day and routines.

Step nine: Determine the next step

Once the data is analyzed, use that information to determine if the interventions should be continued, modified, or terminated.

Data-Based Decision Making

Data-based decision-making is a key component of MTSS. Its overall goal is to improve the quality of education in teaching and learning by allowing schools to

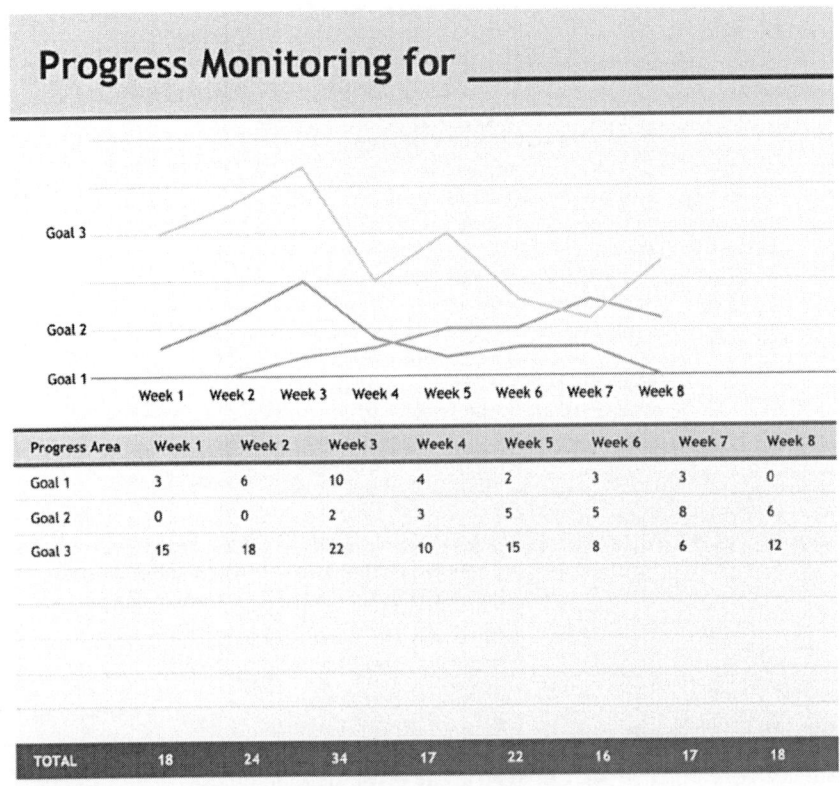

Figure 3.3 Sample progress monitoring chart. Image by author using Microsoft Excel.

allocate resources in ways that enhance student achievement and promote equitable outcomes. Data is collected using a variety of methods, including formal, informal, research data, and big data (Schildkamp, 2019). Table 3.3 outlines the types of data that should be considered when using a data-based decision-making model.

A process known as sense-making allows for the data to be translated and used to inform decisions made regarding interventions. It is important to have key stakeholders involved in the sense-making process because they are the ones who know the students and settings best, and they can provide insight into how data can be translated to meet the needs of the particular population, group, or individual (Schildkamp, 2019). In other words, professional reasoning and intuitive knowledge are key to this process. We will take a closer look at this now.

Table 3.3 Types of Data

Type of Data	Definition	Example
Formal data	Systematically collected uniformly with many different sources, including qualitative and quantitative data	Progress monitoring
Informal data	The information gathered in the day-to-day interactions with students and teachers through observation, conversations, assignments, etc.; sometimes known as professional judgment (Vanlommel & Schildkamp, 2018)	Teacher reports Observations
Research data	The use of published research to inform educational practices; educators will consume published research, analyze its results, adapt the findings to fit the unique needs of their setting and population, and apply that knowledge within their educational context (Flood & Brown, 2018)	Peer-reviewed journal articles
Big data	Big data often comes from large databases gathered across populations; this data is often used to inform policies that impact education	State test scores Health information from major payer sources, such as Medicaid

Sense-Making Process

Initially developed by Karl E. Weick, the sense-making process can be defined as the process of interpreting data while adding new information into an existing framework to guide understanding (Weick, 1995). This means that individuals assign meaning to data based on their own experiences. Progress monitoring involves many members of the educational team collecting and interpreting data. Without sense-making, data gathered from progress monitoring lacks the meaning and context required to make decisions and influence change to support student needs. The process of sense-making involves a collaborative interpretation of data from various perspectives and priorities to synthesize meaningful information (INTRAC, 2017). The education team may rely on a sense-making model to evaluate and process data from progress monitoring and make decisions about supports provided to students at various Tier levels. When interpreting progress monitoring data, school personnel follow the process of sense-making, such as the learning analytics (LA) process model that begins with the implementation of the intervention, gathering data, awareness and reflection of data, and action in response to data (Duval, 2011). By working together as a team and using a process such as sense-making, school personnel can generate informed decisions about the effectiveness of interventions implemented at each MTSS level.

The sense-making process is how occupational therapists can assist in interpreting data within the context of the school environment. It provides guidance for team members, including occupational therapists, to determine factors that contributed to the progress or lack of progress of the students. Progress may be attributed to the support provided, including persons within the environment and environmental support, as well as the traits of the students (Bertrand & Marsh, 2015). School personnel can better understand data in progress monitoring through the sense-making process, helping them to know what interventions to continue, modify, or discontinue.

Occupational therapists are well equipped to assist in the sense-making process within the educational team. Today, many entry-level occupational therapy degrees are at the doctoral level and at least have to be at a master's level. This means occupational therapists have training in the research process, including performing research studies, statistical analysis, interpretation of research data, and implementation of research findings into clinical practice (known as knowledge translation). As part of their entry-level training, occupational therapists read many peer-reviewed research papers and have to provide clinical applications of these studies. They understand that evidence-based practice includes the compilation of research, clinical expertise, and the needs of the client, whether the client is a population, group, or individual.

The process of applying published research to clinical practice is known as knowledge translation. Knowledge translation understands that research is often performed in controlled environments with heterogeneous populations that are not usually seen in the clinical setting. Therefore, there is an understanding that research informs practice and that research must be adapted to inform the clinical decision-making of occupational therapy practitioners to meet the unique needs of their clients in specific settings. According to the FRAME (framework for reporting adaptations and modifications to evidence-based interventions; Wiltsey Stirman et al., 2019), a model developed to track how and why practitioners adapt published research, research may be adapted for many different reasons, including socio-political (laws, regulations, historical context, societal norms, etc.); the policies of the specific district and school; the needs, biases, and person factors of the person implementing the research; and the needs and person factors of the client (population, group, or individual). Decisions regarding adapting evidence are made systematically through a process of consideration of these factors. When adapting evidence, it is important to have clearly defined reasons for what is being modified, why the modification is occurring, and when the modification is taking place (Wiltsey Stirman et al., 2019).

In the school setting, evidence may have to be adapted as many evidence-based interventions have yet to be provided in the school setting. Modifications are often made in a specific and systematic way by practitioners, due to various factors based on the practice setting. In the school setting, it is often social, political, and organizational/environment factors that require the intervention to be adapted. When school-based occupational therapy practitioners understand why interventions are adapted, they are better able to make the best modifications to maintain as much fidelity as possible, while still ensuring the client's needs are met and helping ensure the success of the sense-making process.

When implementing interventions for sensory processing integration in school settings, occupational therapists' suggestions need to be evidence-based and data-driven, and progress needs to be monitored to achieve the best results for their clients. They are also paramount for deciding which tier of support students require.

Deciding on a Tier

Progress monitoring and data-driven decision-making are the foundations for deciding which tier should be implemented to improve and support student learning and positive behavior. Often the occupational therapy team is left out of the decision-making process in Tier 1 and may not even be considered in Tier 2. However, under the Every Student Succeeds Act (ESSA), occupational therapists are identified as specialized instructional support personnel (SIPS) and should be included within every Tier, not only Tier 3. However, many districts may be unsure of how to include occupational therapists within the lower Tier levels, meaning the occupational therapist must advocate for their inclusion. Advocating for inclusion in these Tiers from an organizational level will be discussed in detail in Chapter 8.

Whether or not the district currently includes occupational therapy in the Tier 1 intervention process, the occupational therapist needs to be aware of their role in this Tier. Remember, Tier 1 applies to all students, so occupational therapy should be involved in developing sensory plans, sensory activities, and sensory environments that meet the needs of the population of the school or classroom. In order to provide evidence-based interventions that are tailored to the needs of the population, the occupational therapist should begin by assessing the student population's school environment, routines, and needs. There are certain considerations that may indicate the need for sensory interventions at a population level. For example, if the school is located in a place with limited parks nearby, the occupational therapist may know that students do not have access to playground equipment outside of the school playground. As a result, the students may need additional sensory vestibular and proprioceptive experiences due to lack of access to climbing equipment, swings, and other movement opportunities in their community. It is also crucial to understand the culture of the school. Some schools may value academic time over free play time and limit recess. In a case such as this, the occupational therapist would understand the need to help design Tier 1 interventions to increase movement opportunities without disrupting academic learning time.

CONSIDERATIONS FOR DEVELOPING TIER 1 INTERVENTIONS

- Demographics of the population of the school
  - The average age of parents of students
  - Obesity levels; nutrition/hydration
  - Socioeconomic status
- Access to sensory experiences outside of school
  - Parks nearby
  - Access to extracurricular activities not school-related
  - Family structure and culture of the area as it relates to sensory experiences, namely play experiences and structured movement-based leisure activities
  - Students who walk or bike to school versus those who are driven to school or ride the bus
  - Safety of area related to playing outside
- Importance of movement to the culture of the area
- Routines of the school
  - Number of recesses per day
  - Length of recess
  - Number of physical education classes each week
  - Before and after school programs
  - Other sensory experiences during the school day
- Attitudes of the school personnel
  - Openness to alternative seating arrangements
  - Openness to changing classroom routines and environments
  - Understanding of sensory processing and the impact on learning and behavior
  - Teaching to various learning styles (auditory, visual, kinesthetic)
- Sensory environment of the school and classrooms
  - Auditory
  - Visual
  - Access to movement
  - Access to tactile/proprioceptive experiences

Remember, all students should have access to Tier 1 interventions, so occupational therapists should be assisting school personnel in the development of sensory supports and interventions within a Tier 1 level. Understanding the demographics, values, community, and culture of the school informs the occupational therapist of the sensory needs of the school as a whole as well as individual classrooms.

CONSIDERATIONS FOR DEVELOPING TIER 2 INTERVENTIONS

Typically, students are identified as requiring a Tier 2 level of support through the universal screening process. Through progress monitoring, the occupational therapist can work with other school personnel to interpret data and determine if Tier 1 supports are the best level of support for the student, or if additional, more targeted sensory supports are warranted. For example, through classroom observation or universal screening, the occupational therapist may see that the classroom is responding well to the movement breaks built into the classroom. However, the occupational therapist may identify two to three students that seem to need additional sensory input and are still struggling with calming and organizing, which are required to attend to instruction and follow the routines of the classroom. The occupational therapist can provide additional assessment of sensory processing for identified students (discussed in Chapter 4) to determine their more individualized sensory needs and formulate an additional movement schedule for these students to be implemented with the classroom movement breaks.

Students at the Tier 2 level of intervention have focused and identified needs for additional support. The interventions at this level still need to be considered with Tier 1 interventions, and they should be performed in addition to interventions at the population level. Since students receiving services at the Tier 2 level have identified needs, they can be matched with other students with similar needs. This means that small groups of students with similar sensory processing patterns can allow for more focused interventions. On the other hand, it may be advantageous to group students who have strengths in certain sensory systems with other students who may have strengths in their areas of weakness.

Tier 2 interventions for sensory processing can focus on two main aspects. The first is creating smaller spaces that are conducive to specific sensory needs. For example, occupational therapists can help teachers design areas with low levels of sensory stimulation, such as areas with lower levels of lighting or more sound absorption, and provide a defined area, such as in a corner or with dividers, that students receiving Tier 2 interventions can use for learning. For students with sensory sensitivities, these areas can be used to facilitate increased engagement and participation in classroom work. Additionally, the occupational therapist could create another area with moveable seating and fidgets to allow space for students who need additional sensory input to meet their needs. This space may also have additional visual cues to help students know where to focus their attention.

However, these options for additional input and support should be tailored to the needs of the group of students receiving Tier 2 interventions. With the help of the teacher, the occupational therapist can carry out sensory profile assessments (formal or informal) on the students via a questionnaire or preference checklist. This will help the occupational therapist know which students would

Table 3.4 Quick Small Group Sensory Activities to Support Sensory Regulation

Sensory Needs	Suggested Group Activities in a Short Amount of Time
High need for movement (hyporesponsive to vestibular)	• 10 door jumps – jump 10 times and touch the head of the door frame • 20 windmills – 10 on each side • 30 seconds of bouncing on a large therapy ball Repeat three to five times
Calming	• Using a rocking chair • Wrapping in a weighted blanket • Listening to white noise or calming music Implement for 10-15 minutes during quiet reading time
Motor planning	Simple yoga sequences, such as sun salutation Repeat three times
Proprioceptive and tactile (general organization)	• Bear or crab walk for 15 ft • 10 wall push-ups Repeat three times and follow with arm squeezes or massages on arms and legs

benefit from each space and when they need it, which can then help the teacher structure the day to fit the sensory needs of the students (i.e. organizing the schedule so students have access to different spaces when it is best for them). Of course, under Tier 1 the spaces can be available for all students according to their needs. Under Tier 2, students would have specific times in their schedules when these spaces would be available, and where and when they used them would be based on their sensory profiles.

The second method to address sensory processing differences under a Tier 2 model is to create sensory small groups. These groups can provide specified sensory interventions to address sensory processing needs. Table 3.4 provides some examples of small group activities that address sensory processing needs and can be done in five to ten minutes. These sensory activity sequences may be used to design sensory group interventions for students receiving Tier 2 sensory supports.

Considerations for Developing Tier 3 Interventions

Tier 3 interventions are implemented after the formal referral and evaluation for special education services. Under a true MTSS model, the student would have already experienced Tier 1 and Tier 2 interventions, and more intensified interventions may be warranted when these levels do not provide enough support. Similar to students receiving Tier 2 support, students receiving Tier 3 interventions should also continue to receive interventions at lower Tiers. In this Tier, the student's needs are assessed individually and considered within the environment, and interventions are tailored to the specific sensory needs of that student as outlined in the IEP.

Evidence-based sensory-based interventions in the school setting at a Tier 1 and Tier 2 level that are based on formal or informal assessment data are key to the success of a sensory-based MTSS program. When the occupational therapist is involved in each Tier and when progress monitoring data is uniform and interpreted using a sense-making approach, clear determinations about the need for additional support are easily observed in the data of student progress. Students who have been identified as having additional support needs, even after implementation of Tier 2 supports, may need more individualized plans and interventions. At this point, the occupational therapist should work with the school team to recommend the student for an evaluation for special education services. Remember, occupational therapy is not a stand-alone service under Tier 3, and a student must have identified needs in one of 14 eligibility categories. In addition, to qualify for Tier 3 interventions, which fall under an IEP, students must go through the entire process including evaluation, eligibility, and the establishment of an IEP. The occupational therapist is an important part of the IEP and evaluation team and should consider sensory processing needs as part of the comprehensive assessment. The occupational therapist can include the data from progress monitoring at the Tier 1 and Tier 2 levels in addition to standardized assessments, observation-based assessments, and proxy report assessments to create a clear picture of the student's needs. When the occupational therapy process is followed throughout all Tier levels, including assessment, intervention, and monitoring outcomes, the transition to higher levels of support or to lower levels of support is clearly seen in the data of the student progress.

Tier 3 services are guided by the student's IEP in terms of the method of service delivery and service minutes. However, Tier 3 services should still be embedded in the MTSS model and does not replace the services provided at lower Tiers. Rather these services are in addition to the services already in place to support the student. Occupational therapy practitioners should follow federal, state, and district guidelines for assessment, implementation, and progress monitoring for Tier 3 services.

A Quick Note on 504 Plans

We briefly discussed the difference between an IEP and 504 plan in Chapter 1. Some students may have additional, higher level sensory processing needs that are not able to be adequately addressed at a Tier 1 or Tier 2 level. These students may also have difficulties that do not impact their ability to perform academically. If the student meets other criteria for receiving a 504 Plan, then they may be able to receive individualized occupational therapy services under a 504 Plan to address sensory needs. Each district has different policies and procedures on 504 Plans, but it is important for the occupational therapist to know this is an option for students with higher sensory processing needs that may not qualify for special education.

Summary

The occupational therapy practitioner is responsible for designing and implementing sensory interventions to support academic performance and positive behavior in the school setting. They should assess, plan, and implement sensory interventions at each MTSS level, providing support to other school personnel in the process. The MTSS levels align with the occupational therapy practice as outlined in the OTPF-4, which can serve as a valuable resource for occupational therapists working within various MTSS levels to help define the occupational therapy process within each Tier. Successful implementation of sensory interventions at each Tier level can help support students to succeed within the school setting, and provide required data to support decisions to change levels of support based upon a student's performance and response to intervention. Quality data gathered through assessment and progress monitoring allows the occupational therapist to make evidence-based decisions regarding treatment for clients at each tier to help improve occupational performance for all students at the population, group, and individual levels. In order to effectively gather and implement evidence-based interventions, and develop a plan to track progress according to the effectiveness of the intervention, the occupational therapist must administer high-quality assessments and evaluations. Chapter 4 will review in detail the assessment process at each of the Tier levels with a specific focus on Tier 1 and Tier 2 evaluation, assessment, and outcomes.

Note

1 https://www.cl-asi.org/.

References

American Occupational Therapy Association (AOTA) (2012). *AOTA practice advisory on occupational therapy in Response to Intervention.* https://www.aota.org/practice/practice-settings/-/media/e7371c748756467ba101d6966bb98eb2.ashx.
American Occupational Therapy Association (AOTA) (2020). Occupational therapy practice framework: Domain and process–Fourth edition (OTPF-4). *American Journal of Occupational Therapy, 74*(S2), 1–85. https://doi.org/10.5014/ajot.2020.74S2001.
American Institutes for Research (AIR) (2023). *Essential components of MTSS.* https://mtss4success.org/essential-components.

Ben-Sasson, A., Carter, A. S., & Briggs-Gowan, M. J. (2009). Sensory over-responsivity in elementary school: Prevalence and social-emotional correlates. *Journal of Abnormal Child Psychology*, *37*, 705–716. https://doi: 10.1007/s10802-008-9295-8.

Bertrand, M. & Marsh, J. A. (2015). Teachers' sensemaking of data and implications for equity. *American Educational Research Journal*, *52*(5), 861–893. https://doi.org/10.3102/0002831215599251.

Borkowska, A. R. (2017). Sensory processing disorders–diagnostic and therapeutic controversies. *Current Issues in Personality Psychology*, *5*(3), 196–205. https://doi.org/10.5114/cipp.2017.70140.

Cahill, S. (2019). Best practices in multi-tiered systems of support. In G. Frolek Clark, J. E. Rioux, B. E. Chandler (eds), *Best Practices for Occupational Therapy in Schools*, 2nd ed., pp. 3–10). AOTA Press.

Dean, E. E., Little, L., Tomchek, S., Wallisch, A., & Dunn, W. (2022). Prevalence models to support participation: Sensory patterns as a feature of all children's humanity. *Frontiers in Psychology*, *13*, 875972. https://doi: 10.3389/fpsyg.2022.875972.

Duval, E. (2011, February). Attention please! Learning analytics for visualization and recommendation. In Proceedings of the First International Conference on Learning Analytics and Knowledge, pp. 9–17. https://doi.org/10.1145/2090116.2090118.

Dweck, C. S. (2010). Can we make our students smarter? *Education Canada*, *49*(4), Canadian Education Association.

Flood, J. & Brown, C. D. (2018). Does a theory of action approach help teachers engage in evidence-informed self-improvement? *Research for All*, *2*(2), 347–358. https://doi.org/10.18546/RFA.02.2.12.

Garwood, J. D. & Ampuja, A. A. (2019). Inclusion of students with learning, emotional, and behavioral disabilities through strength-based approaches. *Intervention in School and Clinic*, *55*(1), 46–51. https://doi.org/10.1177/1053451218767918.

INTRAC (2017). *Sensemaking*. https://www.intrac.org/wpcms/wp-content/uploads/2017/01/Sensemaking.pdf.

Jussila, K., Junttila, M., Kielinen, M., Ebeling, H., Joskitt, L., Moilanen, I., & Mattila, M. L. (2020). Sensory abnormality and quantitative autism traits in children with and without autism spectrum disorder in an epidemiological population. *Journal of Autism and Developmental Disorders*, 50, 180–188. https://doi.org/10.1007/s10803-019-04237-0.

Law, M., Cooper, B., Strong, S., Stewart, D., Rigby, P., & Letts, L. (1996). The person-environment-occupation model: A transactive approach to occupational performance. *Canadian Journal of Occupational Therapy*, *63*(1), 9–23. https://doi.org/10.1177/000841749606300103.

Lopez, S. J. & Louis, M. C. (2009). The principles of strengths-based education. *Journal of College and Character*, *10*(4). https://doi.org/10.2202/1940-1639.1041.

Mulligan, S., Douglas, S., & Armstrong, C. (2021). Characteristics of idiopathic sensory processing disorder in young children. *Frontiers in Integrative Neuroscience*, *15*, 647928. https://doi.org/10.3389/fnint.2021.647928.

Schildkamp, K. (2019). Data-based decision-making for school improvement: Research insights and gaps. *Educational Research*, *61*(3), 257–273. https://doi.org/10.1080/00131881.2019.1625716.

Vanlommel, K. & Schildkamp, K. (2018). How do teachers make sense of data in the context of high-stakes decision making? *American Educational Research Journal*, *56*(3), 792–821. https://doi.org/10.3102/0002831218803891.

Watling, R., Miller Kuhaneck, H., Parham, L. D., & Schaaf, R. (2018). *Occupational Therapy Practice Guidelines for Children and Youth with Challenges in Sensory Integration and Sensory Processing*. AOTA Press.

Weick, K. E. (1995). *Sensemaking in Organizations*, 3rd ed., pp. 1–231. Sage Publications.

Wiltsey Stirman, S., Baumann, A. A., & Miller, C. J. (2019). The FRAME: An expanded framework for reporting adaptations and modifications to evidence-based interventions. *Implementation Science*, *14*, 1–10. https://doi.org/10.1186/s13012-019 -0898-y.

Chapter 4

Assessing the Need for Sensory Interventions

Introduction

As we explored in Chapter 3, student sensory needs can be addressed at all levels under a multi-tiered system of supports (MTSS) model, as guided and monitored by the occupational therapy practitioner. Now, in this chapter we will deepen our knowledge further by looking at how we assess the need for sensory interventions at various MTSS levels. We will begin by providing an overview of what assessment and evaluation are, and then move on to outlining the importance of carrying out assessments before implementing sensory interventions. After detailing formal and informal assessment methods, we will review best practices for assessing both population level and small group level. To conclude, we will examine how to gather quality data and produce high-quality reports to develop effective interventions for those in need. As Tier 3 assessments are traditional to occupational therapy services in school settings, and are well-known to most occupational therapists, the majority of the chapter will discuss assessments at Tier 1 and Tier 2 levels.

Overview of Evaluation and Assessment

The occupational therapy process always begins with an evaluation, which consists of the occupational profile, an analysis of occupational performance, and a synthesis of the evaluation (American Occupational Therapy Association [AOTA], 2020). Evaluations are what the occupational therapist uses to identify the client's strengths and areas of decreased occupational performance, and to develop individualized treatment plans to address client-centered goals. The evaluation is an ongoing process that begins with the initial interaction with the client, and the purpose is to determine the needs and wants of the client, what the client has done and can do, define supports and barriers, and identify what well-being and participation mean to the client (AOTA, 2020).

You can see an example of an occupational therapy sensory motor evaluation in Figure 4.1. This sample evaluation includes the occupational profile,

DOI: 10.4324/9781032654768-5

Sample Occupational Therapy Evaluation

Occupational Profile:
>   Developmental/Medical History
>   Strengths
>   Supports
>   Barriers
>   Goals for Therapy

Fine Motor/Gross Motor:
>   Standardized Fine/Gross Motor Test
>   Clinical Observations Related to Fine and Gross Motor Skills

Range of Motion/Tone:
Motor Stability/Postural Control:
Balance and Equilibrium Reactions:

Sensory Processing/Modulation:
>   ***Standardized Assessment of Sensory Reactivity***

>   Assessment/Clinical Observations of Sensory Integration and Processing:
>   - Vestibular processing
>   - Ocular motor/visual processing
>   - Bilateral integration
>   - Projected action sequences
>   - Proprioceptive processing
>   - Tactile processing
>   - Auditory processing
>   - Motor planning and sequencing

Self-Care:

Summary of Findings:
>   Section One: Draw conclusions regarding fine motor, postural control, motor stability strengths and functional deficits.

>   Section Two: Discuss sensory modulation/reactivity and discrimination abilities in each sensory system.

Figure 4.1 Sample occupational therapy sensory motor evaluation. Image by author.

assessment of motor skills, assessment of sensory processing, assessment of self-care, summary of findings, and an intervention plan.

From this, it is no surprise that assessment goes hand-in-hand with evaluations as another key part of occupational therapy. Crucially, assessment identifies the need for occupational therapy services, defines the strengths and areas of concern for clients, and provides information to develop a holistic, skilled, and client-centered intervention plan. This could look like interviews, records reviews, proxy reports, standardized assessments, non-standardized assessments, and observations.

Due to policies dictating the evaluation of student needs, when working in the school setting it is important for us to understand the difference between evaluation and assessment. Assessments are methods that we use to gather data on the client as part of the evaluation process. Some primary methods could include reviewing current available information, such as educational, developmental, and medical history. As we will explore throughout this chapter, the data collected should be from various sources and be multidisciplinary. This is so we create a complete picture of the student beyond just their occupational history.

On the other hand, evaluation is part of the occupational therapy process and initiates the implementation of occupational therapy services. Let us take a closer look at this process together.

Evaluation Process Under IDEA

Evaluation is an essential part of IDEA, which is explored fully in Chapter 1. As occupational therapists, this is what we use to determine a student's eligibility for special education services. This occurs when a child has been identified as needing more individualized help under Tier 3 after Tier 1 and Tier 2 interventions have shown that they do not provide enough support for the student.

Under IDEA, parents must be informed of the evaluation and its process before the evaluation is initiated. Naturally, the input from the parent or caregiver of the child is key to the evaluation, and many districts require written permission from the parent or guardian before this process can begin. The permission signed by the parent or guardian must outline the aim of the evaluation and the procedures the evaluation team will use to assess the child for a disability.

So, what is the aim of these evaluations? This evaluation process aims to determine if the child has a disability that is impacting their performance in the school setting. Importantly, it should also provide information on the services an eligible student would need to be successful in a school environment. For best practice, the evaluation process must use a variety of assessment methods (i.e. at least two) to examine the child's development, academic performance, and functional performance, and, in short, to determine if the child is eligible for more specialized support. For example, a speech-language pathologist may provide evaluation data to determine if a student is eligible for speech-language impairment. As considered best practice, two assessment methods should be used to gain data, and then these assessments can be compared to provide a more complete picture of the child's level of functioning. To ensure the accuracy of these assessments, it is essential that the following criteria are met.

- The assessment methods used during the process are sound instruments and have good reliability and validity without bias.
- The assessments should be provided in the student's native language, by trained personnel, and in the manner they were intended to be used.
- A multidisciplinary team should perform the evaluation and assess any area of suspected disability.
- The evaluation must be comprehensive to ensure all of the student's needs or potential needs are assessed.
- Areas should not be assessed only if they are related to the suspected disability. Rather, any area of special education or related services that may impact a child's performance in school should be part of the evaluation process (Individuals with Disabilities Education Act, 2017).

Box 4.1 is an example of this in action.

BOX 4.1   CASE EXAMPLE: SARAH

Sarah is a second grade student who has always done well in school. However, she began to struggle about halfway through the first quarter of her second grade year. Her performance was slipping and she was not at grade level for reading. She began to struggle to pay attention during seated desk work and often got in trouble for talking or being out of her seat. She also began to have difficulty with other students and had even gotten in trouble for hitting and kicking other students. Because of her difficulties with behavior and academics, Sarah was referred for Tier 2 interventions for positive behavioral support and reading. However, after six weeks, progress monitoring showed a decrease in Sarah's reading performance and an increase in behavioral referrals. Therefore, she was referred for a multidisciplinary evaluation to determine eligibility for special education instruction under Tier 3 services. After receiving signed permission from Sarah's parents, the team initiated assessments in the following areas.

- Psychological testing consisting of intelligence testing, behavioral assessment, and adaptive skills assessment.
- Academic testing in reading and math.
- Speech-language testing consisting of two language assessments, assessment of articulation, and assessment of pragmatic language.
- Occupational therapy testing consisting of fine and gross motor assessment and assessment of sensory integration and processing.

The Occupational Therapist's Role in Evaluating Sensory Processing

The evaluation of sensory processing should be included in any occupational therapy evaluation for a student with a suspected disability. While sensory processing differences are commonly related to the disabilities outlined in IDEA, such as autism, the assessment of sensory processing should not be limited to just this disability category. Since occupational therapy is a related service, the occupational therapist is often part of different student evaluations, and many students with disabilities may have sensory processing differences that impact their educational performance.

When assessing sensory processing, the occupational therapist must provide proper evaluations to identify if a student has sensory processing differences. From this, it is necessary to determine whether or not those differences impact the student's ability to participate in school activities and perform academic-related tasks. This means that occupational therapists should assess sensory processing using a variety of methods, and that they must also assess participation. Therefore, assessment methods of sensory processing should not only be observer-reported outcomes, but also performance-based assessment methods that can be combined with observer-reported measures. For example, an occupational therapist can use the Sensory Processing Measure-2 (SPM-2) (Parham et al., 2021), which is a common teacher-reported assessment of sensory modulation and reactivity.

To combine this with an example, let us return to Sarah from the case in Box 4.1. As part of the occupational therapy evaluation, the occupational therapist provided Sarah's teacher and parents with an electronic version of the SPM-2 to complete. This assessment is a proxy-report measure that tends to focus on identifying sensory reactivity issues. A school form was provided to Sarah's teacher to see how her sensory reactivity impacted her school performance. A home form was provided to Sarah's parents to examine how Sarah's sensory processing looked in the home environment.

However, to get a full picture of the student, this should not be the only assessment utilized to determine if a child has sensory processing differences that impact educational participation. An occupational therapist should also employ a performance-based evaluation, such as the Structured Observations of Sensory Integration-Motor (SOSI-M) (Blanche et al., 2021), the Goal-Oriented Assessment of Life Skills (Miller et al., 2013), or the Evaluation of Ayres Sensory Integration (EASI) (Mailloux et al., 2018). Returning to Sarah, the occupational therapist decided to utilize the SOSI-M to further examine Sarah's sensory processing and integration beyond just reactivity. The occupational therapist wanted to see how Sarah was processing and integrating sensory input to generate motor responses needed to perform her school-related tasks. The SOSI-M coupled with the SPM-2 afforded the occupational therapist the ability to draw conclusions about Sarah's sensory systems, identify her sensory strengths, and note areas that lead to participation challenges for Sarah in the school setting.

If standardized assessments of sensory processing and integration are not available, or if the occupational therapist does not have the adequate training to administer and interpret performance-based sensory assessments, such as the EASI, the occupational therapist should perform structured observations to determine if sensory processing needs are impacting participation in academic-related tasks. If the occupational therapist observes any sensory processing challenges, they should link this to any impacts on participation. However, it is important to recognize that the presence of sensory processing differences does not necessarily mean that they impact the student's ability to participate in school activities. This process of linking sensory processing and participation will be discussed later in this chapter.

Next, we will explore why it is integral that occupational therapists conduct evaluations before providing interventions at any MTSS level.

Evaluation Before Providing Interventions

Occupational therapists are frequently consulted in the school setting regarding sensory interventions for individuals and the classroom. Mostly, these interventions include sensory-based interventions and environmental modifications. However, as best practice, these interventions should be implemented by an occupational therapist, and should not be implemented at all without an evaluation taking place first. But, why is this the case?

Firstly, it has to be the occupational therapist who issues the implementations because they are the experts in sensory integration and processing. The role of the school-based therapist is multi-faceted, and the occupational therapist's role is to assist by making recommendations for universal design for learning. As occupational therapists, we have the knowledge and training to evaluate sensory integration and processing, understand how sensory processing impacts participation in school activities, and provide skilled interventions to increase student occupational performance. While other school personnel may have knowledge of sensory processing and integration, the occupational therapist is the only professional who understands the range of ways sensory integration and processing can occur, how it impacts learning, the interaction between the person and the environment, and how to design sensory interventions to facilitate participation.

Additionally, it is best practice for occupational therapists to collect assessment data before implementing any interventions. This can be seen from The American Occupational Therapy Association's series, where they highlight best practice recommendations. One of these recommendations addresses sensory-related interventions and how occupational therapy practitioners should implement these intervention strategies. The recommendation states the following.

> Don't provide sensory-based interventions to individual children or youth without documented assessment results of difficulties processing or integrating sensory information.

(AOTA, 2024)

This best practice recommendation assures two things. First, it outlines and determines that occupational therapists are the professionals who should be providing sensory-based interventions. It indicates that the occupational therapist has the training and expertise to provide these interventions, that sensory-based interventions are part of the occupational therapy scope of practice, and that sensory needs should be managed by occupational therapy practitioners, not other personnel.

Second, it provides guidance on how assessment should occur before the implementation of sensory interventions. This allows the occupational therapist to assess children before providing interventions, which is part of the occupational therapy process. It also prevents the occupational therapist from providing global sensory recommendations that do not match the needs of the client without assessing and documenting the need for the intervention. This allows the occupational therapist to ensure interventions are skilled and can only be provided by someone with sensory integration and processing expertise.

It puts an end to the situations that occur in the school setting where teachers and other professionals ask the occupational therapist for sensory equipment and recommendations without the occupational therapist knowing the student, or whether or not the student has sensory processing needs. For example, other professionals may approach the occupational therapist requesting a weighted vest or noise-canceling earphones for a student. If the occupational therapist has not provided some level of assessment, even if just an interview or observation, they should not provide the sensory equipment. Without assessing, providing sensory-based interventions may be at best ineffective or at worst harmful to the student. When assessment occurs, the occupational therapist can provide the type of sensory input or sensory environmental modification that meets the child's unique sensory processing needs. If sensory-based interventions do not increase participation, they should not be utilized.

In addition to the initial assessment, this best practice recommendation supports occupational therapists in monitoring the progress and success of sensory-based interventions. The occupational therapist is skilled at linking areas of need to participation in order to provide interventions that increase participation, not just provide support for sensory processing needs. As sensory needs and the sensory environment change, the occupational therapist should monitor and assess the provided intervention for effectiveness and modify the intervention as needed as it impacts participation in the different school settings.

Proximal and Distal Outcomes in Sensory Integration and Processing

The evaluation process of sensory processing and integration can be complex and cumbersome. Although this text does not seek to provide an exhaustive description of how to assess and interpret sensory evaluation data, it will present some common principles that the occupational therapist must be aware of when administering an evaluation.

Occupational therapists may utilize a top-down or bottom-up approach to assessment and intervention. Often the occupational therapist will utilize both approaches. When using a top-down approach, the occupational therapist first evaluates, focusing on participation and engagement, and considering a range of factors that may impact the client's participation. Under this approach, sensory integration and processing are considered, but only as part of the participation process as a whole. Examples of assessment tools utilized in a top-down approach include the Canadian Occupational Performance Measure (COPM) (Law et al., 2019). While the occupational therapist considers the client factors and performance skills, the main focus of evaluation is participation.

In a bottom-up evaluation approach, the occupational therapist focuses on performance skills and client factors, and they consider how these areas impact the participation of the client. Under this approach, sensory processing is evaluated as part of the client factors. Hypotheses are formulated as to how the client factors of sensory integration and processing impact participation and engagement in daily tasks. Regardless of the approach, the goal of the occupational therapy practitioner is to improve participation in the chosen occupations.

Proximal Outcomes

In sensory integration and processing, the occupational therapist evaluates both proximal and distal outcomes. Proximal outcomes are a client factor, and they relate to how the body processes sensory information (Schaaf et al., 2015). Under the Occupational therapy practice framework: Domain and process–Fourth edition (OTPF-4) (AOTA, 2020), sensory functions are classified as a body function under client factors. These include visual, hearing, vestibular, taste, smell, proprioceptive, and touch functions, interoception, pain, and sensitivity to temperature and pressure. In contrast to proximal outcomes being how the body processes sensory information, distal outcomes are how sensory processing impacts participation (Schaaf et al., 2015).

Occupational therapists frequently assess sensory functions from a reactivity and modulation standpoint. They may use questionnaires in tandem with performance-based assessments to help understand how sensory reactivity impacts participation in various environments. Table 4.1 provides examples of standardized assessments that can be used to evaluate sensory reactivity and modulation.

Table 4.1 Sensory Reactivity/Modulation Assessments

Assessment Name	Forms for Children of School Age	Environments
Sensory Processing Measure-2 (SPM-2) (Parham et al., 2021)	Preschool (2–5 years) Child (5–12 years) Adolescent (12–21 years)	School form
Sensory Profile 2 (Dunn, 2014)	3–14 years	School companion
Sensory Experiences Questionnaire (Baranek et al., 2006)	2–12 years	One form
Evaluation in Ayres Sensory Integration® (EASI) (Mailloux et al., 2018)	3–12 years	Child report; not specific to an environment

Occupational therapists should also assess sensory processing beyond modulation and reactivity. This is because the assessment of sensory processing and integration can provide needed information about motor planning, sequencing, coordination, postural control, balance reactions, and ocular motor control, which are all areas that can impact a child's ability to perform educationally relevant occupations. The other important aspect of evaluating sensory integration and processing is to provide information on whether sensory integration and processing are part of the underlying cause of barriers to participation or if another factor may be causing the barrier. In other words, sensory processing and integration assessment can "rule out" sensory issues as they relate to participation or confirm that sensory processing and integration are part of why the client is having difficulties.

The evaluation data provides the information the therapist needs to make those decisions. Many children may exhibit similar difficulties in participation, but one child's difficulties may be related to sensory processing, while another child's difficulties may be related to a different area, such as cognition. The assessment process determines the underlying cause of these barriers to participation and allows the occupational therapist to develop a treatment plan to address these difficulties. In other words, the occupational therapist links underlying areas of difficulty to difficulties in occupational performance, thus providing information as to where intervention should occur.

Because of their training and expertise in sensory processing, the occupational therapist needs to be the one who assesses sensory processing and integration. Other members of the multidisciplinary team may identify potential sensory processing difficulties, but the occupational therapist is the team member who is trained to differentiate how the underlying cause is related to sensory processing challenges. The process of doing this requires skilled evaluation and observation skills, and the occupational therapist must consider each factor that may be causing difficulties in participation in school-based occupations. The occupational therapist will more than likely also perform standardized assessments.

Performing standardized assessments provides data on whether the child is performing as would be expected of other children of the same age. Coupling standardized assessments with observational data and questionnaires and/or interviews with the student, teacher, caregivers, and other personnel can help paint a complete picture of the child's performance and identify where barriers to participation may be occurring. The occupational therapist should consider sensory factors, other client factors, and the environment when deciding whether sensory integration and processing are creating a mismatch between the child's performance and expectations. If it is determined that sensory processing and integration are barriers, then sensory interventions would be warranted. Sensory interventions may be direct, indirect, or changes to the sensory environment. This will be discussed in detail in the next chapter.

Performance-Based Assessments

It is common in the school setting for occupational therapists to utilize teacher-report questionnaires as a main part of the evaluation process for students with suspected sensory processing differences. While questionnaires are important, they only present one viewpoint, especially when they are observer-reported outcomes. In addition, most of the standardized teacher-report and even self-reported assessments of sensory processing are not designed to measure outcomes and progress. Too often, the only standardized assessment of sensory processing is a teacher-reported measure, such as the SPM-2 or SP2, with no further assessment of sensory processing and integration.

However, while proxy report measures of sensory processing are important, it is not enough to take only reported information and make adequate determinations about the impact of sensory processing on school performance. The occupational therapist should also ensure that other assessment methods are utilized to fully understand the client in that environment, such as performance-based assessments of sensory processing, sensory integration and motor skills, and participation. Table 4.2 provides some common performance-based assessments that can be used to assess sensory integration and processing. In addition to direct performance assessments, the occupational therapist needs to ensure that the student's voice is heard. The student's perception and report of their own strengths, barriers, and sensory processing is key to provide a full picture of the student within the school setting.

Table 4.2 Performance-Based Assessments of Sensory Integration and Processing

Assessment	Ages	Areas of Sensory Integration and Processing Assessed
Evaluation in Ayres Sensory Integration® (EASI) (Mailloux et al., 2018)	3–12 years	Balance Postural control Coordination Sequencing Praxis Ocular motor Projected action sequences Modulation/reactivity and discrimination
Structured Observations of Sensory Integration-Motor (SOSI-M) (Blanche et al., 2021)	5–14 years	Balance Postural control Sequencing Coordination Ocular motor Projected action sequences Proprioception
Bruininks-Oseretsky Test of Motor Proficiency–Third Edition (BOT-3) (Bruininks & Bruininks, 2024)	4 years, 0 months–25 years, 11 months	Balance Postural control Sequencing Coordination Projected action sequences
Goal-Oriented Assessment of Life Skills (GOAL) (Miller et al., 2013)	7–17 years	Projected action sequences Coordination Postural control Praxis

Assessment of Transitions Between Tasks and Activities

Many students need help with transitions between classroom activities and between different environments in the school setting. Children with transition difficulties often have sensory processing differences that contribute to their challenges in managing transitions effectively, causing disruption and distress for the student and other members of the class. The occupational therapist can be crucial in determining the best intervention method for students who are struggling with these transitions, offering tailored sensory supports to help increase participation.

Method of Evaluation

One important aspect of assessing transitions is using observation and interview evaluation methods. The occupational therapist should observe the classroom routines at several intervals throughout the day and on different days of the week. They observe to determine the frequency and consistency of transitions, how the transition is indicated, the smoothness of the transition, and whether the students are engaged during the transition process. The time of the transition should also be noted, as well as any supports the students need to complete the transition (i.e. verbal prompts or direction, visual cues, large group instructions, individual instruction, etc.). The occupational therapist should also observe if peers assist any students in the transition process or if the observed students transition independently. Specifically related to sensory processing, the occupational therapist needs to note what type of activities occur directly before students have difficulties with transitions. This is because the type of sensory input in activities directly preceding the transition may impact the transition. For example, students with problems transitioning from music class to the general education classroom may have auditory sensitivities that cause their nervous system to be in a higher state of alertness, making it difficult for them to attend to classroom tasks. They may be seeking out input to organize, which disrupts their ability to transition smoothly to the classroom environment.

To help with these observations, the occupational therapist should ask the teacher for a copy of the daily schedule with transition times noted. As the

Table 4.3 Evaluating Transitions

Criterion	Observed	Partially Observed or Observed with Support	Not Observed
Student starts tasks promptly upon instruction			
Transitions between activities/ environments are smooth			
Minimal to no disruptions during routine activities			
The student demonstrates an understanding of routine expectations			
Students help each other transition between tasks			
The teacher provides clear instructions and reminders as needed			
Transitions are completed within the expected timeframe			
The student needs additional support from the teacher to complete the transition			
The student needs additional time to complete the transition			

observations occur, the occupational therapist must note any behavioral incidents and disruptions within the transition. In addition, the occupational therapist should discuss academic performance with the teacher to monitor any correlations with the current classroom routines and flow. It is also important to include the students in the evaluation of transitions. By asking the students how they feel about routines and how their body feels during transitions, you are provided with helpful insights into why a student may be experiencing difficulty. It can also provide information on whether or not sensory supports may help students transition.

Table 4.3 is a chart to help guide observations and evaluations of transition observations. This chart can be modified to meet the needs of your environment.

Distal Outcomes

As previously mentioned, proximal outcomes are related to how the body and brain process and use sensory information. On the other hand, distal outcomes are associated with the participation of the students in the school setting (Schaaf et al., 2015). In other words, proximal outcomes relate to sensory processing, such as hyporeactive to vestibular input, whereas distal outcomes relate to participation, such as how a student moves about the classroom during large group instruction. Proximal and distal outcomes should be linked as the goal of occupational therapy is to improve participation. When proximal outcomes are not clearly linked to distal outcomes of occupational performance and participation, the occupational therapist is at risk of focusing on symptom reduction rather than on facilitating participation.

Priorities for distal outcomes are determined by the student, parents or caregivers, teachers, and other members of the educational team. Occupational therapists should consider distal outcomes of all aspects of the school day from academic and behavioral perspectives. Often it is evident that sensory sensitivities are the causes for difficulties in participation due to students avoiding tasks or becoming distracted by sensory stimuli. However, recent research shows that hyporeactivity to sensory input is associated with behavior that impedes learning and negatively correlates with behaviors that facilitate learning (Marchum & Tavassoli, 2024). It may be very evident when a student is avoiding activities due to hyperreactivity to sensory input, but the occupational therapist must be mindful to assess reactivity from both hyperreactivity and hyporeactivity and determine if any sensory processing difference may be impacting participation in classroom and school-related activities. By performing a thorough assessment, the occupational therapist can link sensory reactivity to participation in school activities.

Table 4.4 provides some examples of how the proximal outcomes of sensory processing relate to distal outcomes of participation in school occupations.

Table 4.4 Sensory Outcomes and School Tasks

Sensory System	School Tasks
Vestibular processing	Sitting upright in a chair or on the floor
	Maintaining seated positions
	Standing in line
	Grasping a pencil
	Cutting with scissors
	Reading (ocular motor control)
	Copying from the board or a worksheet
Proprioceptive processing	Grasping a pencil or other objects
	Walking down the hallway and staying in line
	Performing fine motor tasks accurately such as writing and coloring
Tactile processing	Being in groups of students (standing next to others in line, seated near others on the floor)
	Writing, coloring, typing
	Using manipulatives
	Keyboarding
	Sensory play
Auditory	Following directions
	Attending to quiet work
	Social participation with peers
Visual	Reading
	Writing, cutting, drawing, coloring
	Following routines

Most available assessments look at either proximal outcomes or distal outcomes of sensory processing. Few sensory assessments link proximal outcomes to distal outcomes, and very few link sensory processing to participation, specifically in the school setting. It is the role of the occupational therapist to draw conclusions and link proximal assessment data to distal assessment data. However, an assessment is available that specifically examines participation and the sensory environment within one measure. It is known as the Participation and Sensory Environment Questionnaire–Teacher Version (PSEQ–TV)[1] (Piller, 2017).

This assessment provides an overview of how the sensory environment impacts participation in various preschool classroom activities. It is reliable and valid (Piller et al., 2017) and can be used as a screening tool or as part of a more comprehensive evaluation. Figure 4.2 provides a sample of the scores generated from the assessment, with higher scores indicating increased difficulties with participation. These activities with higher scores highlight where the occupational therapist should design interventions to either support the sensory environment or the sensory processing of the client to improve the fit between the person and environmental demands.

PSEQ-TV Raw	0
Circle/Large Group Time Raw	0
Table Time Raw	0
Snack/Lunch Time	0
Classroom Routines	0
Free Play/Recess	0
Craft/Art Time	0
Self Care	0
Movement/Music Time	0
Subtest1: Activities	0
Subtest2: Support	0
Subtest3: Modifications	0

Figure 4.2 Sample scores from PSEQ–TV. Image by author.

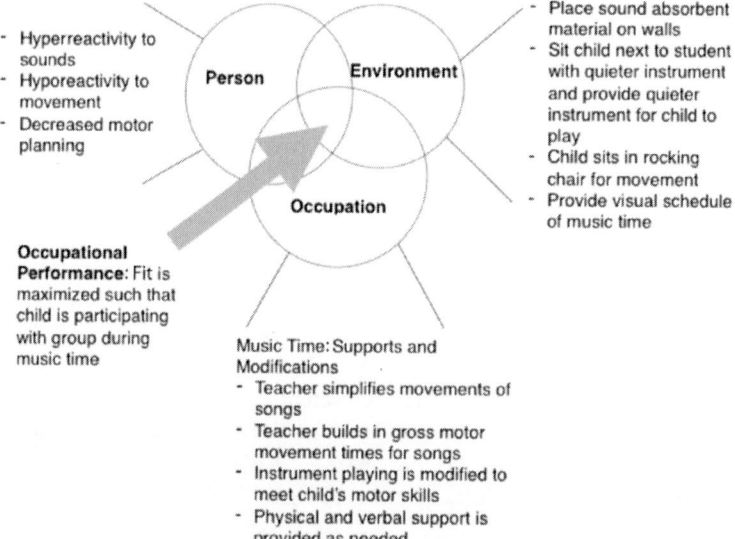

Post-Intervention: Maximized Fit Between Person, Environment, and Occupation

- Hyperreactivity to sounds
- Hyporeactivity to movement
- Decreased motor planning

Person

Environment

Occupation

- Place sound absorbent material on walls
- Sit child next to student with quieter instrument and provide quieter instrument for child to play
- Child sits in rocking chair for movement
- Provide visual schedule of music time

Occupational Performance: Fit is maximized such that child is participating with group during music time

Music Time: Supports and Modifications
- Teacher simplifies movements of songs
- Teacher builds in gross motor movement times for songs
- Instrument playing is modified to meet child's motor skills
- Physical and verbal support is provided as needed

Figure 4.3 Using PSEQ-TV to design interventions (Piller, 2016; used with permission from Aimee Piller).

Teachers frequently coordinate sensory environmental modifications that should be done in collaboration with the occupational therapy practitioner. The PSEQ-TV provides a valuable tool to help design modifications that meet the needs of students as related to specific areas of participation. By using the PEO theory, the environment can be modified to improve the fit of the person and sensory environment to increase participation in various tasks. Figure 4.3 provides an example of pre- and post-intervention using the PSEQ-TV to guide the process under the PEO theory.

Components of Occupational Therapy Evaluation

The occupational therapy evaluation consists of several different components that create a full picture of the client and their needs for occupational therapy services. The entire process is outlined in the OTPF-4 (AOTA, 2020). Let us take a look at the core components together.

Occupational Profile

The occupational profile identifies the rationale for occupational therapy services. It includes the reason for the referral to occupational therapy, outlines the concerns of the client, family, or teacher, and provides background information. The occupational profile is how the occupational therapist gains information about the client's daily routines, occupations, history, feelings of success, and the client's priorities. There are many ways that occupational therapists can gather this information about the client, whether the client is a population, group, or individual. A records review is an excellent way to gain information before meeting the client. It allows the occupational therapist to know what they may need to prepare for the client before the initial meeting. At the population level, a records review may consist of a review of the school's mission, the demographic information of students and staff, and an examination of the policies and procedures of the district. At the group level, a records review may include examining the students' records, including their state assessment scores, current grades, and other relevant background or developmental and learning history. Interviews and observations are also vital to gathering information about the client's occupational profile.

The occupational profile serves many purposes. One of the main reasons for the occupational profile is to determine the areas of importance to the client. This helps the occupational therapist know what occupations and contexts are most important to the client and determine which aspects are supportive and which are hindrances to the client's desired occupational performance. At the population level, this information can be gathered based on the priorities of the district and school. Information on what is important to the district and school can be gathered by reviewing the mission statement of the school and/or district and by examining the priorities of the district, school, and classroom. Ideally, the occupational therapist would have an opportunity to engage in conversation with the key stakeholders of the school, including the school board, administration, and parents. This is not always feasible due to time constraints and access to these individuals. Still, the occupational therapist can view information on the website, attend school board meetings, and even send out surveys. In addition, school board minutes are public information and can be reviewed to help the occupational therapist ensure they are aware of the priorities of the district. Attending special education department meetings, attending school-wide meetings, and engaging in discussions with classroom teachers during their planning period can allow opportunities for the occupational therapist to gain more information about the client's occupational profile at the population level. At the group level, discussion with group members can be an excellent and efficient way to gather information about supports, barriers, and what is important to the client. A focus group format or the use of games can help students feel more comfortable in sharing their occupational profiles.

The occupational profile at the population level often involves a needs assessment. A needs assessment is designed to identify gaps between what is currently happening with a population and what is desired, ultimately pinpointing the reason for seeking occupational therapy services. A needs assessment also provides information on what occupations the population engages in on a regular basis, examines the history of the school and students, and can identify the values and interests of the population by talking with administrators, parents, and other stakeholders of the school or classroom. Needs assessments are performed in a series of steps.

1) Identify the question and target audience. In this case, the question is: What is the school's occupational profile?
2) Develop questions. Questions may include the following.
   a) What is the school's mission statement?
   b) What are the demographics of the students and families in the school?
   c) What are the values and priorities of the school district and administration?
   d) What are the needs of the school?
3) Collect information internally and externally.
4) Analyze and use data to generate an occupational profile.
                                                          (Team Asana, 2024).

Other assessment methods include surveys, forums, focus groups, and interviews. This information can be used to generate a community profile that outlines the needs, values, and perspectives of the school or classroom as a whole.

The occupational therapist gathers information for the occupational profile at the group level by interviewing the group members. Since the group is significantly smaller than the population, the occupational therapist can use many of the same methods of gaining information for the occupational profile as is done at the individual person level. It is important to interview and engage with group members and support personnel, such as teachers and aides, who may be group members at times but not directly in the service group.

Table 4.5 Occupational Profile

Occupational Profile Component	Definition
Reason for Seeking Services	Why the Client is Seeking Services
Perceived success in occupations	What occupations the client feels successful in performing, and what areas impact those occupations they do not feel successful in performing
Occupational history	Past experiences
Values and interests	Values and interests of the client
Context	Determine supporting and inhibiting environment and personal context
Performance patterns	Habits, roles, routines, and engagement in occupations
Client factors	Values, body functions, and body structures that are viewed as supporting or inhibiting
Client goals	The desired outcome of services

Table 4.5 outlines the requirements for an occupational profile per AOTA (2021).

When gathering information about the occupational profile of the population, the occupational therapist can often learn from administrative staff and information provided about the mission and purpose of the school and classroom. Interviewing teachers and principals can also help gather information about the occupational profile of the school, class, and small groups. In addition, exploring the values and needs of the classroom can provide important information about the needs, preferences, and patterns of the population.

When gathering information about a group, the occupational therapist can utilize games to learn more about the group members – for example, icebreaker activities that can be modified to include questions related to the occupational profile. In Box 4.2, you can see some examples of icebreaker games that can be modified and used as part of best practice.

BOX 4.2   GAMES TO GATHER OCCUPATIONAL HISTORY AT THE POPULATION OR GROUP LEVEL

Human Bingo

Create bingo cards with questions from an occupational profile, such as questions that focus on participation in leisure or play activities, goals for the school year, places they have traveled, etc. Each square on the bingo card should contain a characteristic or trait someone might have. For example, "I went to overnight camp this summer," "I enjoy playing sports such as baseball and basketball," and "My goal for the school year is to get good grades." Distribute the cards to each student, making sure the

---

cards are unique so that not everyone will try to get bingo the same way. Tell the students their goal is to mingle and find other students who have the same characteristics on their cards. As they move around the room and talk to one another, they should put the student's name on the square that matches a characteristic. Once a bingo is achieved, the students can bring their cards up for a prize. The occupational therapist can collect the cards and see which students have particular interests, values, and experiences to develop their occupational profile.

Two Truths and a Lie

In this game, each student will write down three statements related to an occupational profile, such as what they enjoy doing, a place they have gone, what is important to them, where they have lived or currently live, etc. Two should be true, and one should be made up. Each student should share their information in any order. After they share, other students guess which is the made-up statement. Students can ask questions to gain more information and determine which statement is made up. Once all students have guessed which statement is untrue, the student speaking can reveal the false statement. The game continues until all students have shared. During this time, the occupational therapist can take notes on information related to the students to complete the occupational profile.

Who am I? Drawing Activity

Provide the students with blank pieces of paper and crayons or markers to draw a picture. Explain that they will be creating a visual representation of themselves, including their identity, interests, personality traits, values, experiences, and where they live. Give them 10–15 minutes to complete the drawing task. Encourage students to be expressive and creative. They can add words or sentences to their drawings as well. Here are some prompts to use to encourage them to add to their drawings.

- What are some words or phrases that describe you?
- What are your favorite hobbies?
- What activities do you like to do outside of school?
- Who are some important people in your life?
- Where do you live? Are there other places that are important to you?
- What emotions do you experience?
- What do you do well at in school?
- What do you wish you had more help with at school?
- What is the hardest part of the school day?
- What is your favorite part of the school day?

In each of these activities, the occupational therapist can use games to facilitate social interactions and self-reflection while gathering information about the occupational profile of more than one student. The occupational therapist can examine the responses and convert them into a comprehensive occupational profile that describes the population or group as part of the Tier 1 and Tier 2 occupational therapy evaluation. Using games can help students engage and feel more comfortable sharing information in a non-threatening manner. It allows the occupational therapist to gain information about the occupational profile quickly and efficiently, while supporting social development and providing opportunities for the occupational therapist to observe the interrelationships within the population and groups.

Evaluation of Occupational Performance

After the occupational profile, the next step of the evaluation process is to assess occupational performance. The information gained from the occupational profile provides the evaluating therapist with the necessary information to determine what type of assessments to perform. Yet, the occupational therapist must also consider the context and how occupational performance may vary in changing contexts and environments. This is especially important when working at an MTSS Tier 1 and Tier 2 level. Specifically in the school setting, the occupational therapist must consider the contexts of the classrooms, playground, lunchroom, hallways, and other settings where students participate in educational-related occupations.

While it may seem difficult to assess occupational performance of a population (Tier 1), it only requires a shift in thinking. The profession of occupational therapy does not currently have many standardized or formal assessments of population-based occupational performance; however, there are many effective, qualitative methods of evaluation that provide rich data if performed rigorously, such as observations and interviews. Observations should capture the elements of the environment, and the routines and performance of the persons within the environment. Interviews can be more focused on providing targeted information on specifics of the sensory environment and occupational performance at designated places within the routine of the school day. In addition, the occupational therapist can focus interview questions on specific sensory systems to gain more specific information about the sensory processing of the class or school as a whole.

Observations

Observations are a form of qualitative inquiry that provide detailed information on the environment as well as the roles and routines of the individuals within

Table 4.6 Components of Observations

Component	Essential Information
Time of observation	• Start time • End time • Total time of observation • Date of observation
Setting	The description of the setting can be a narrative or a drawing/picture • Location of the observation • Description of physical environment • Description of sensory environment • Number of persons in the room • Roles of persons (i.e. students, teachers, aides, etc.) • Arrangement of furniture
Specific data related to the purpose of observation	Specific data should be related to the purpose of the observation • Routines • Roles • Reaction of people to stimuli • Timing and type of stimuli • Task behaviors (when and how often) • Cues provided (how often and when)
Description of events	• Include a sequential description of events • Include persons involved in events • Tell a story of the observation • Be descriptive

the context. They are incredible at giving a full picture of the sensory processing patterns of the school or classroom. In addition, they offer an opportunity to assess occupational performance as it occurs when performing various occupations. For observational data to be helpful to the occupational therapist, they should provide a clear picture of the environment and what happened within the environment, while also noting the client's responses and actions within the environment (Patton, 2015). The key components that should be included in every observation are shown in Table 4.6.

Figure 4.4 provides a sample observation form that can be used by an occupational therapy practitioner to perform classroom observations. The form has open areas rather than lines so that the observer can use text or pictures to document the observations. Box 4.3 provides a sample of an observation performed in a school setting for a middle school student in science class.

School Observation

Name of Student: _____

Date of Observation: _____ Time of Observation: _____

Location of Observation: _____

Observer Name and Credentials: _____

Description of Environment (Physical and Social):

Observations:

Figure 4.4 Sample observation form. Image by author.

BOX 4.3   SAMPLE OBSERVATION WRITE-UP

School Observation

Name of Student: Charlotte S.

DOB: 03/13/2012

Location of observation: Jackson Middle School Science Class

Date of observation: 09/09/2024

Time: 2:15–2:45 PM

Observer: Aimee Piller OTR/L

Description of environment (physical and social):

The room was an average-sized classroom with four rows of tables. Each row had four tables in it with two students at each table. Charlotte was seated in the front row near the teacher's desk at the end table. Her aide was seated on her right side. The classroom did not have any windows. There were two bulletin boards on each of the side walls. The back of the room had a storage area, bookshelves, and two sinks. The front of the room had a regular whiteboard and smart whiteboard.

Observation Notes:

Charlotte was observed seated at her desk in math class. She was sitting in the middle of the classroom. She was seated at a desk/table with one other student and an aide sitting next to her. There were students sitting around her. She was observed wearing headphones and chewing on the lanyard around her neck. Her feet were in the chair. There was an aide sitting near her. The aide was writing something on the paper on Charlotte's desk. Charlotte was observed to fidget with her lanyard and rock in her chair. She was then observed playing with her fingers on her desk (for example, tapping, etc.). The aide gave Charlotte the pencil and cued her to write. The aide then took the pencil back and gave Charlotte a highlighter. The aide took turns with Charlotte writing and highlighting, although the aide appeared to do the majority of the writing. Charlotte was observed to rub her head and pull and twist her hair. She was again observed to rock in her chair. She was observed to write parts of the notes while the teacher was giving a lesson. She then waved her arms in the air. The teacher played a video and Charlotte appeared to be attentive to the video. The aide then cued her it was time to transition and Charlotte began to gather her things. Charlotte was observed to rock in her chair on four occasions during the observation. The aide also gave Charlotte 13 cues for attention.

Impressions:

Charlotte appeared to be overstimulated, which was evident by her frequent rocking, twisting of hair, fidgeting and mouthing the lanyard, and decreased attention. She required frequent cues for attention, and the aide appeared to be doing more than half of the writing for the assignment/notes, rather than Charlotte following along and participating in the assignment. Although she was in the classroom with other students, she demonstrated decreased participation in the classroom tasks. She required frequent cues for attention and only engaged in the work and classroom tasks when cued or assisted by her aide.

Interviews and Focus Groups

The purpose of an interview is to obtain information about a specific event, person, or setting. They allow the occupational therapist to gain valuable insight into the needs of the students. Since you can speak with students directly, interviews can open a window into the student's perspective that cannot be grasped simply through proxy reports (Roberts, 2020). However, it takes a skilled interviewer to ask the right questions to gain the best information and keep the interviewee on topic (Patton, 2015). It is incredibly important that the interview remains objective and free from bias and emotion as much as possible. The goal of the interview is to gather relevant data without focusing on the feelings of the persons involved, which can cloud the results and interventions eventually chosen. Therefore, the interview questions should be open-minded and worded in a way that does not lead the interviewee to answers, and the interviewer must be careful to put aside any assumptions or presumptions about the interviewee and situation.

The first step in interviewing is to develop questions that target the concepts the interviewer wants to have a deeper understanding of. When gathering information about the sensory processing of the school, classroom, or group, interview questions should focus on three main components: sensory processing preferences, the sensory environment, and routines. These interviews can take place with teachers and other school personnel as well as students. Providing core and follow-up questions can allow the interviewer to gain more information about the topic and facilitate more conversation among the interviewees. Interviews provide an excellent opportunity to gain information from the student's perspective rather than just proxy reports (Roberts, 2020). Focus groups are a great way to interview multiple people at one time, allowing individuals to share feedback with a group in a dynamic but moderated manner. Questions for focus groups can be the same as for interviews, but the facilitator must be aware of group dynamics and the need to facilitate participation of all group members, not only a select few that may tend to dominate the conversation.

Once questions for interviews or focus groups have been developed by the occupational therapist or occupational therapy team, the next step is to pilot the questions through a process known as cognitive testing. Cognitive testing helps ensure questions are worded in a way that gathers the intended information. This step ensures that the questions are understood and determines if any changes to the wording of questions need to be made or if any questions should be added or removed entirely. To do this, it is best to ask other occupational therapists or school personnel to review the questions and ask questions about their understanding. Here are some sample questions to ask when conducting cognitive testing for interview questions.

- What does this question mean to you?
- Was the wording of any questions confusing?
- Were there any questions you did not understand?

After receiving feedback from experts, you should modify the questions as needed to ensure understanding and intent. Once questions are well worded, the occupational therapist will want to consider how many questions to ask. It is important to remember that teachers and students are busy, so interviews should be brief. Fifteen to twenty minutes should be sufficient to gather information without requiring too much time from the occupational therapist or interviewee.

BEST PRACTICE FOR INTERVIEWING

It can be difficult to conduct an interview confidently while also obtaining the critical information you need. Some general advice for interviewing is included below, along with some sample questions, to support you when interviewing in school-settings.

1. The occupational therapist should **practice the interview questions ahead of time to make sure they flow in order**.
2. The interview should begin with an introduction and explanation of the purpose of the interview.
3. The occupational therapist should **understand the questions and their intent so that they can reword the question accurately if needed**. It is good practice to have alternative wording of questions prepared beforehand and have a written definition of what specific terms mean in the questions.
4. You should **prepare probing questions to gain more information**. Some interviewees may want to share a lot of information, and the challenge here will be keeping them on topic. In contrast, others may require additional probes and examples to share even minimal information.
5. To begin, you should **build rapport with the interviewee** so they are comfortable sharing information and their feelings during the interview. This may include explaining your role in the school setting and asking a few personal questions about the person.
6. **Be mindful of the interviewee and their time**. It is important to make sure the interviewee has time for the interview, giving them an estimate of how long the interview might take. You should also make sure the environment is relaxed and quiet.
7. **Be attentive when listening**. It is important to restate information if needed to ensure accuracy of understanding. People appreciate it if you show them that you are genuinely listening to their answers. You can do this by asking follow-up questions for clarification or providing examples if the person seems to have trouble thinking of an answer to the question. Looking at the person and providing affirmative but non-judgmental nonverbal feedback, such as nodding, can help the person answer more thoroughly.
8. **Take thorough notes during the interview and, if necessary, record the interview** if the person provides permission. Make sure to inform the person you will be taking notes ahead of time, so they do not feel you are not listening to them.

BOX 4.4   SAMPLE INTERVIEW QUESTIONS

- Describe a typical day in your classroom.
- When do you feel the students perform the best during the day? When do you feel the students have the most difficulties during the day?
- What is your biggest concern regarding the students?
- What do you think is the class's greatest strength this school year?
- What does sensory processing mean to you? How do you consider sensory needs in your classroom?
- What sensory activities do you currently use? When do you use them? Are they effective?
- What is your goal for this school year? What would you like to see your students accomplish? What support would help you reach that goal?
- What do you feel works best in your classroom to help students stay on task?
- How do students respond during transition time? Do they need support? Is this an easy time of day or more chaotic?

Surveys

A benefit of interviews is that they can easily be turned into surveys to save time and allow more participants to provide feedback. The process for developing survey questions should follow the same process as interview questions.

First, the occupational therapist should clearly identify the reason for the survey by stating the question that should be answered by the data collected. This will keep the survey questions targeted to this topic. Next, they need to develop questions related to the topic. In contrast to questions asked during an interview, these questions should be more specific rather than open-ended. Although you can make survey questions open-ended by including text boxes for longer responses, this may require increased time for analysis and completion by the participants. Instead, using Likert scales allows participants to easily and quickly identify priorities, needs, and current levels of occupational performance. Likert scales can be in the form of ratings, satisfaction, quality, frequency, performance, importance, and focus (Kusmaryono et al., 2022). If open-ended questions are used as part of the survey, analysis should be performed via narrative analysis methods, either through reading and analyzing text or using artificial intelligence to assist with analyzing recurrent themes.

Survey questions should also go through the process of cognitive testing before distribution to ensure questions are written and understood as intended. Having one or two occupational therapists review the surveys ahead of time can ensure the questions are written in a way that is clear, true to the intention, and free from grammatical errors.

The next step is to load the survey into the desired online platform for ease of distribution. Many different types of survey software are available for free (i.e. Google Forms), and some school districts may have access to other paid survey software (i.e. Qualtrics). It is essential to familiarize yourself with the software's features and ensure surveys are only accessible to identified personnel or students for the identified amount of time. Once the survey is closed, the data can be analyzed and reported as part of the assessment process. Most of the survey platforms synthesize the data collected to provide a summary of data that can easily be interpreted and put into a report.

Questionnaires

Many questionnaires are available to evaluate sensory processing, the sensory environment, and the school and classroom routines. Some questionnaires are standardized, whilst others are informal questionnaires designed to gather more general information. Some districts may classify these questionnaires as part of the formal assessment process, and therefore they would require parental permission before administering and would be more appropriate to provide when evaluating Tier 3 eligibility and needs. This would mean parental permission would be required before administering these questionnaires. Table 4.7 provides some examples of standardized questionnaires that may be used in the home or school setting, depending on which version is used.

Informal questionnaires are readily available online or can be created by the occupational therapist. They are an easy and affordable way to examine the specific needs of the setting and are manageable for students and school personnel.

Table 4.7 Sensory Questionnaires

Name of Assessment	Area Assessed
Sensory Processing Measure-2 (SPM-2) (Parham et al., 2021)	Person factors – sensory processing
Sensory Profile 2 (SP2) (Dunn, 2014)	Person factors – sensory processing
Participation and Sensory Environment Questionnaire– Teacher Version (Piller, 2017)	Sensory environment
Classroom Sensory Environment Assessment (C-SEA) (Kuhaneck & Kelleher, 2018)	Sensory environment

They are also often considered screening tools and, therefore, can be part of the universal screening process rather than deemed a formal assessment method.

Direct Assessment of Performance

Direct assessment of skills and occupational performance is standard, especially at the Tier 3 level of intervention, and tends to be more focused on the specific needs of an individual child. However, direct assessment at the Tier 1 and Tier 2 levels is also important for occupational therapists. Assessing direct performance at the population and group levels provides a method of evaluation to determine what areas of occupational performance are being impacted by sensory processing. It also allows the occupational therapist to identify strengths to tailor interventions toward the client's strengths.

When assessing the group and population levels, the occupational therapist still examines a person's impact on the group and population. It may be easy to identify students with sensory processing challenges when performing population and group assessments, but the occupational therapist must be skilled to ensure they do not shift their focus to evaluate that individual. They need to continue to evaluate the population and group, knowing that the individual they may particularly notice impacts the performance of the population and group. To help stay focused on the group, it may be helpful to keep a list of performance skills being observed, namely motor, processing, and social interactions (AOTA, 2020).

The goal of the evaluation is to examine the members of the group or population and how they impact the function of the group and the population as a whole. For example, if an individual within a reading group is off task and getting up and down from their seat, this may impact the engagement of the entire group in the reading and comprehension of the story. The occupational therapist would note the performance of the group but indicate that one group member's performance impacted the functioning of the group as a whole.

The Evaluation of Sensory Integration and Processing

A full evaluation of sensory processing consists of the components of an occupational therapy assessment as described above and outlined in the OTPF-4. As explored, the evaluation should include formal and informal assessment methods, evaluation of sensory modulation, evaluation of sensory discrimination, evaluation of postural, ocular, oral, and bilateral motor control, assessment of motor skills, assessment of praxis, assessment of organizational skills, and how sensory integration impact performance and participation (Parham et al., 2011). Specifically, when conducting the more objective measures of sensory processing, the occupational therapist should assess sensory processing (reactivity and modulation) via observation, performance assessment (as detailed in Table 4.2), or questionnaires (i.e. SPM-2, SP2). In addition, sensory integration should be assessed to determine if motor planning, sequencing, postural control, and visual skills are impacted. An evaluation of motor skills, routines, behavior, and social-emotional factors should also be included in a full evaluation. This allows the occupational therapist to link assessment results of sensory processing and integration (proximal outcomes) to occupational performance in the areas of participation in academic tasks, interaction with others, adherence to routines, and completing daily activities (distal outcomes). The occupational therapist should synthesize and assess all of the information to clearly define how a client is processing sensory information and how that impacts performance within the school setting. If the results are clearly linked, the treatment plan is easy to establish and implement.

So far, this chapter has considered how assessments should be conducted from the perspective of an occupational therapist, gathering the input of caregivers, teachers, and other school personnel. Now, let us turn to how we can consider and incorporate the child's perspective into our assessments for supports and interventions.

The Child's Perspective in Assessment

Many sensory processing assessments in pediatrics are from the perspective of the teacher or caregiver, who report on the child's sensory processing based on the frequency of observed behaviors. As children get older, there are more self-report measures of sensory processing that often accompany a teacher or caregiver reported questionnaire. However, just because a child is younger does not mean that their perspective should not be considered. In fact, the student's perspective is essential to the evaluation process and should not be ignored. The caregiver and teacher perspective are important, but they do not actually assess feelings of the child, who experiences the sensory processing. Many sensory processing assessments only provide information on how frequently the child reacts or does not react in a certain way. While valuable information, it does not reflect what the child actually feels or experiences in sensory processing. When the child's perspective is not considered, the child may feel unsupported or disrespected (Söderbäck et al., 2011).

The occupational therapist can utilize many methods to gain the child's perspective for their assessment, such as through interviewing. When interviewing students, it is crucial to ask questions that match their level of cognitive and language understanding. By asking simple questions about how certain activities make them feel or what activities help them learn, you can obtain valuable information that helps you understand the child's perspective of their sensory processing. Another way this can be achieved is by using questionnaires that are designed or modified for younger children so they can provide insight on their own sensory processing. The occupational therapist should consider the developmental level of the child and modify questionnaires as needed to ensure the child understands the question and is able to provide a response reflective of their perspective. Using pictures or allowing for gestures rather than verbal or written answers can also help allow non-speaking students to share their thoughts and feelings as part of their assessment of sensory processing.

The Sensory and Satisfaction Questionnaire, developed by Stansberry & Piller (2023), is a tool that allows children as young as three years of age to provide input on how they process sensory information and their satisfaction with therapy services. It was developed as part of a quality improvement study at a pediatric therapy clinic and piloted on over 100 clients to determine its feasibility. Below are some examples of the questionnaire for various age levels.

BOX 4.5   *SAMPLE OF THE SENSORY AND SATISFACTION QUESTIONNAIRE* BY AMBER STANSBERRY AND AIMEE PILLER

Pre-K Questions Sensory

1. I like looking at shiny or spinning things (Example: fidget spinners).
2. I like playing in a dark room (Example: a room with no lights on).
3. I like bright lights (Example: if seated in a well lit area can state, "A room with all the lights on like where we are sitting right now.").
4. I get scared or upset when I hear loud sounds (Example: the sound of thunder during a storm or a vacuum cleaner).
5. I like being in crowded or busy places (Example: restaurants, grocery stores, the big gym, etc. This means places where there are a lot of people around me).

Elementary

Look at the picture below. There is a happy face and a sad face. The happy face means yes and the sad face means no. For all of the questions I am going to ask you, you can either tell me yes or no or point to one of the faces. Are you ready to start?

Elementary Questions Sensory

1. I like looking at shiny or spinning things (Example: fidget spinners).
2. I like playing in a dark room (Example: a room with no lights on).
3. I like bright lights (Example: if seated in a well lit area can state, "A room with all the lights on like where we are sitting right now.").

4. I get scared or upset when I hear loud sounds (Example: the sound of thunder during a storm or a vacuum cleaner).
5. I get distracted by background noises (music, family or classmates talking, fans, etc.) when I am doing my schoolwork or homework.

Figure 4.5 shows a sample answer key from the assessment. Answers include "yes," "somewhat," and "no" matched to a smiley face, small smile face, and frown.

1) Yes   2) Somewhat   3) No

Figure 4.5 Sample responses from Sensory and Satisfaction Questionnaire. Image used with permission.

By gaining the child's perspective, the occupational therapist can better understand the child's needs and tailor interventions to those needs. Combining the child's perspective with the caregiver's and teacher's perspective can help provide a more holistic picture of the child's sensory needs, occupation preferences, and participation in occupations.

Synthesis of Evaluation Data

The final step in the evaluation process for occupational therapists is to synthesize the evaluation data. In the assessment of sensory processing and integration, this involves linking proximal to distal outcomes. Sensory integration and processing data should be synthesized as a proximal outcome, describing the child's sensory processing, including strengths and areas that may need improvement. The documented evaluation report should comment on the sensory processing of the individual, group, or population, depending on what client was being evaluated. Let us take a look at this process together.

First, the evaluation summary should include a summary of the client's performance skills, specifically related to sensory processing. This includes the

Table 4.8 Chart for Tracking Sensory Processing by System

Sensory System	Hyper	Hypo	Expected Range	Discrimination	Not Observed
Visual					
Auditory					
Tactile					
Vestibular					
Proprioception	-				
Olfactory					
Gustatory					
Interoception					

proximal data from evaluations (formal and informal) and should comment on how the client processes sensory information, including reactivity (hyper, hypo, or within expected range), sensory discrimination (no significant issues or difficulties with discrimination), and sensory-based motor performance (including postural control, balance, ocular motor, coordination, and motor planning). Each sensory system should be addressed so that adequate interventions can be generated. Table 4.8 demonstrates how this can be achieved without missing a key consideration.

Once sensory processing has been determined, the synthesis should include a summary of how the environment impacts occupational performance. The assessment should comment on the facilitators within the environment, meaning what aspects of the sensory environment support performance, and the barriers within the environment, meaning the aspects of the sensory environment that hinder occupational performance.

Finally, the synthesis of the evaluation should link the client factors of sensory processing to the environmental factors in order to draw conclusions on the performance skills of the client. This is where the occupational therapist summarizes how the client's sensory processing and the sensory environment impact the client's performance. Sensory processing can impact motor skills, other performance skills, and the process of performance, including the organization of space, time, and objects, and social interactions. When utilizing a sensory integration frame of reference, the occupational therapist considers these the proximal outcomes. The idea is that the occupational therapist provides a clear link between the sensory processing of the client (proximal) and the performance skills that result in occupational performance (distal). Box 4.6 provides an example of a synthesis for a client at the person level and group level.

BOX 4.6   PERSON LEVEL

Meredith appeared to be registering vestibular input, which was evident by post-rotary nystagmus (PRN) within the average range. Meredith presented with decreased proprioceptive processing impacting her ability to perform accurate movements. Difficulties with vestibular and proprioceptive processing impacted Meredith's postural control, balance, ocular motor skills, and coordination. Although she appeared to be registering vestibular input, Meredith had a high threshold for vestibular input, meaning she may need additional movement throughout her day to regulate and organize. Meredith's tactile discrimination fell in the above-average range. Other tactile assessments also fell within the average range. She was very aware of tactile input and demonstrated the ability to discriminate between tactile input. However, she tended to be more on the hyperreactive side to tactile input. This may have been causing her nervous system to be in a state of high alert much of the time. As a result, she may have to use cognitive energy to calm and organize, and attend, thus impacting her ability to attend and complete daily tasks, or she may seek out vestibular and proprioceptive input to calm her nervous system. She did not appear to have any hyper reactivity [sic] to auditory input.

With motor planning (praxis), Meredith demonstrated difficulties with postural praxis and had significant difficulties with imitating body positions. Difficulties with somatosensory processing can impact motor planning as information regarding body positions is not registered or interpreted to correct motor positions. Children with motor planning difficulties may rely more on cognitive strategies to reason through motor plans. Novel motor tasks and familiar motor tasks performed in a variant manner may have been difficult for Meredith to perform independently. As a result, Meredith may have avoided certain tasks, attempted to control an activity or task to ensure success, or tended towards the same task repeatedly.

Meredith's difficulties with sensory processing may have impacted her ability to organize and calm throughout the day to complete her academic tasks and follow classroom routines.

GROUP LEVEL

The group was composed of six students with sensory processing needs in the areas of vestibular, proprioceptive, and tactile. The students presented with hyporeactivity in vestibular, proprioceptive, and tactile areas, causing them to seek out additional sensory input during classroom activities that should be more sedentary. The main times of the day when the students would seek additional input were after lunch, specials, and recess. This indicated that during these times, they were able to get some of their sensory needs met but did not get to their sensory threshold and needed additional sensory input to regulate and organize to attend to classroom activities. The increased need for sensory input caused the students to seek out additional input such that their ability to complete classroom activities was limited.

Consideration of Outcomes

Occupational therapists are tasked with identifying outcomes from the onset of the evaluation, and it is important to consider their purpose. The individualized education program (IEP) goals frequently measure progress and effectiveness of provided interventions for students receiving services under a Tier 3 model. A similar approach can be used in Tier 1 and Tier 2 through progress monitoring. The goals should be written in such a way that they are measurable and attainable within an expected time frame. The SMART goal is the standard method for writing goals in the educational setting (Doran, 1981). Each letter of SMART stands for a component of the goal.

- **Specific**: Includes specifics of what should be accomplished, who is involved, where it will take place, why it is important.
- **Measurable**: Includes criteria for measuring progress and determining when the goal has been achieved.
- **Achievable**: Realistic and attainable within a given time frame and with available resources.
- **Relevant**: Aligns with broader objectives and long-term goals of the student.
- **Time-bound**: Has a clear timeframe for completion.

Occupational therapists may also consider other methods of developing outcomes. For example, if looking at the environment, the occupational therapist can complete a second observation or interview and compare results from the initial assessment to the follow-up assessment to see if changes have been made. Also, many school districts have established methods for progress monitoring. These methods must be considered when establishing outcomes to align with expected school and district goals and can be an effective tool to assess outcomes of occupational therapy interventions.

When choosing an outcome measure, occupational therapists must consider the intervention they want to assess. The aim is to determine if the support and intervention provided is successful in reaching the set goals, and then decide whether to continue, modify, or terminate the intervention. Therefore, the outcome measure selected should be a tool or method that is able to determine change. Questionnaires related to sensory reactivity, such as the SPM-2 or SP2, are not designed to measure progress since sensory reactivity varies daily and in various environments. Instead, occupational therapists should consider measures of participation to determine if participation has improved. To choose the best outcome, occupational therapists should consider the purpose of the goals and make sure this is clearly defined in how the goal impacts participation in the school environment.

They should also consider which domain, such as physical, cognitive, social, or emotional, is relevant. It is important to remember that sensory processing is not the domain that should be considered. Rather, the occupational therapist should consider how sensory processing impacts physical, social, emotional, and other domains. Each setting has different available measures, so it is essential to consider what assessment methods are available and can be used within the expected time constraints of the therapist. Above all, the occupational therapist should ensure that the outcome measure aligns with the client's goals, intervention plan, and context. If standardized assessments are used, the psychometric properties, specifically test-retest reliability, should be considered when choosing a standardized assessment to demonstrate effectiveness.

Summary

Regardless of which tier of MTSS the occupational therapy practitioner is working under, the first step in the occupational therapy process is assessment and evaluation. Assessments and evaluations provide information on what a client needs to participate in daily occupations. Evaluation can occur at the population, group, and client level and should include formal and informal assessment methods. While this can take some creativity from the occupational therapist, it is an essential first step before interventions are developed. Through the evaluation process the occupational therapist understands the client strengths and barriers and is able to tailor the intervention plan to meet the unique needs of the client in the school setting. They do this by identifying how sensory processing (proximal outcomes) impacts participation in the school setting (distal outcomes). When evaluation is performed properly, the intervention plan and methods of tracking progress are clear, targeted, and effective. Without proper evaluation, there is no way for any school personnel to know the needs of the students at any level. Providing sensory interventions without an evaluation is not effective, nor is it an efficient use of anyone's time. But, when proper assessment occurs, interventions are matched to the client's needs, at each MTSS level. It takes the guesswork out of designing interventions and instead provides concrete data to guide and track sensory interventions.

In Chapter 5, we will discuss how to use assessment data to design evidence-based sensory interventions that can be used in the school environment at all MTSS levels to build on strengths, decrease barriers, and support participation of students with sensory processing needs.

Note

1 Available for free at https://participationandsensoryenvironment.weebly.com/pseq--
   -teacher-version.html.

References

American Occupational Therapy Association (AOTA) (2024). *An update on AOTA's best practice recommendations (formerly Choosing Wisely®).* https://www.aota.org /practice/practice-essentials/evidencebased-practiceknowledge-translation/aotas-top -10-choosing-wisely-recommendations.

American Occupational Therapy Association (AOTA) (2021). Improve your documentation and quality of care with AOTA's updated occupational profile template. *American Journal of Occupational Therapy*, 75 (S2), 7502420010. https:// doi.org/10.5014/ajot.2021.752001.

American Occupational Therapy Association (AOTA) (2020). Occupational therapy practice framework: Domain and process–Fourth edition (OTPF-4). *American Journal of Occupational Therapy*, *74*(S2), 1–85. https://doi.org/10.5014/ajot.2020.74S2001.

Baranek, G. T., David, F. J., Poe, M. D., Stone, W. L., & Watson, L. R. (2006). *Sensory Experiences Questionnaire (SEQ).* APA PsycTests. https://doi.org/10.1037/t07997 -000.

Blanche, E. I., Reinoso, G., Kiefer, D. B. (2021). *Structured Observations of Sensory Integration-Motor (SOSI-M).* ATP Assessments.

Bruiniks, B. D. & Bruininks, R. H. (2024). *Bruininks-Oseretsky Test of Motor Proficiency–Third Edition.* Pearson.

Doran, G. T. (1981). There's a SMART way to write management's goals and objectives. *Management review, 70*(11).

Dunn, W. (2014). *Sensory Profile 2.* Pearson Assessments.

Individuals with Disabilities Education Act (IDEA) (May 3, 2017). *Sec. 300.304 evaluation procedures.* https://sites.ed.gov/idea/regs/b/d/300.304.

Kuhaneck, H. & Kelleher, J. (2018). *Classroom Sensory Environment Assessment (C-SEA).* Academic Therapy Publications.

Kusmaryono, I., Wijayanti, D., & Maharani, H. R. (2022). Number of response options, reliability, validity, and potential bias in the use of the Likert scale education and social science research: A literature review. *International Journal of Educational Methodology*, *8*(4), 625–637. https://doi.org/10.12973/ijem.8.4.625.

Law M., Baptiste S., Carswell A., McColl M. A., Polatajko H. J., Pollock N. (2019). *Canadian Occupational Performance Measure*, 5th ed., revised. COPM Inc.

Mailloux, Z., Parham, L. D., Roley, S. S., Ruzzano, L., & Schaaf, R.C. (2018) *Evaluation in Ayres Sensory Integration® (EASI).* n.p.

Mailloux, Z., Parham, L. D., Roley, S. S., Ruzzano, L. & Schaaf, R. C. (2018). Introduction to the evaluation in Ayres Sensory Integration® (EASI). *American Journal of Occupational Therapy, 72*, 7201195030p1–7201195030p7. https://doi.org /10.5014/ajot.2018.028241.

Marcham, H. & Tavassoli, T. (2024). Relationship between directly observed sensory reactivity differences and classroom behaviors of autistic children. *American Journal of Occupational Therapy*, *78*(3), 7803345010. https://doi.org/10.5014/ajot.2024 .050345.

Miller, L. J., Oakland, T., & Herzber, D. S. (2013). *Goal Oriented Assessment of Lifeskills (GOAL™)*. Western Psychological Services.

Parham, L. D., Ecker, C. L., Kuhaneck, H., Henry, D. A., & Glennon, T. J. (2021). *Sensory Processing Measure, Second Edition (SPM-2)*. Western Psychological Services.

Parham, L. D., Roley, S. S., May-Benson, T. A., Koomar, J., Brett-Green, B., Burke, J. P., Cohn, E. S., Mailloux, Z., Miller, L. J., & Schaaf, R. C. (2011). Development of a fidelity measure for research on the effectiveness of the Ayres Sensory Integration® intervention. *American Journal of Occupational Therapy*, *65*(2), 133–142. https://doi .org/10.5014/ajot.2011.000745.

Patton, M. Q. (2015). *Qualitative Research & Evaluation Methods* (4th ed.). Sage Publications.

Piller, A. (2017). *The participation and sensory environment questionnaire–Teacher version*. https://participationandsensoryenvironment.weebly.com/pseq---teacher-version.html.

Piller, A. (2016). *The reliability of the sensory environment and participation questionnaire–Teacher version*. [Doctoral Dissertation, Texas Woman's University.]

Piller, A., Fletcher, T., Pfeiffer, B., Dunlap, K., & Pickens, N. (2017). Reliability of the participation and sensory environment questionnaire: Teacher version. *Journal of Autism and Developmental Disorders*, *47*, 3541–3549. https://doi.org/10.1007/ s10803-017-3273-3.

Roberts, R. E. (2020). Qualitative Interview questions: Guidance for novice researchers. *Qualitative Report*, *25*(9). https://doi.org/10.46743/2160-3715/2020.4640.

Schaaf, R. C., Cohn, E. S., Burke, J., Dumont, R., Miller, A., & Mailloux, Z. (2015). Linking sensory factors to participation: Establishing intervention goals with parents for children with autism spectrum disorder. *American Journal of Occupational Therapy*, *69*(5), 6905185005p1–6905185005p8. https://doi.org/10.5014/ajot.2015 .018036.

Söderbäck, M., Coyne, I., & Harder, M. (2011). The importance of including both a child perspective and the child's perspective within health care settings to provide truly child-centred care. *Journal of Child Health Care*, *15*(2), 99–106. https://doi.org/10 .1177/1367493510397624.

Stansberry, A. & Piller, A. (2023). *The Sensory and Satisfaction Questionnaire* [Unpublished Assessment].

Team Asana. (2024, February 23). What is a needs assessment? 3 types and examples. *Asana*. https://asana.com/resources/needs-assessment.

Chapter 5

Designing Interventions to Address Sensory Processing Needs

Introduction

Throughout this book, we have explored in depth how sensory processing can impact a student's ability to learn in the school setting. As part of the occupational therapist's role in promoting accessible education for all, we have looked at the importance of understanding how our different sensory systems can cause students to react differently to their school environment, and what methods occupational therapists can use to assess and evaluate what interventions are needed at Tier 1 and 2 levels. Now, this chapter will describe how occupational therapists can interpret assessment data to generate treatment interventions that address sensory processing needs in the school setting. It will provide several examples of interventions for the Tier 1 and Tier 2 levels that focus on the sensory environment and the client's sensory processing, providing practical suggestions on what interventions to use, and how to implement them within classroom routines.

Sensory Processing Patterns

As discussed in the previous chapter, assessment is the first step of the occupational therapy process. The occupational therapy assessment aims to identify the client's strengths and weaknesses with two primary goals. First, it establishes and justifies the need for occupational therapy services, and second, it provides information to develop a treatment plan to achieve client-centered goals and improve occupational performance and participation (American Occupational Therapy Association [AOTA], 2020). Occupational therapists are skilled at summarizing information from an evaluation to generate a profile of the client, whether the client is a population, group, or individual. This process involves identifying strengths, areas of concern, barriers to participation, and reasons these barriers exist. The summary should provide an overview of the client, the client's goals, and the client's current level of functioning.

DOI: 10.4324/9781032654768-6

Unlike other related therapy disciplines, such as physical therapy and speech-language pathology, occupational therapists do not provide formal diagnostic evaluations. However, occupational therapists still follow a similar process of identifying areas of concern and patterns that align with certain diagnostic categories. This is especially true in the evaluation of sensory integration and processing.

When evaluating sensory integration and processing, the occupational therapist formulates a hypothesis and performs evaluation techniques to prove or disprove the hypothesis. Under a traditional Ayres Sensory Integration® (ASI), the occupational therapist will assess each sensory system as to how it reacts to sensory stimuli to determine if there are any signs of hyperreactivity, hyporeactivity, or processing within adequate or expected range. As explained in Chapter 2, when a child displays hyperreactivity to sensory input, otherwise known as over-responsive or hyperresponsive, this means that the intensity of stimuli it takes to elicit a response is less than what is expected, often resulting in an adverse response to sensory stimuli. On the other hand, when a child is hyporeactive to sensory input, which is also known as under reactive or hyporesponsive, the child appears indifferent to sensory input and requires more sensory stimuli or more intense sensory stimuli than expected to elicit a response. These children may display more seeking or craving behaviors toward sensory input, meaning that they tend to engage in tasks and activities that provide high levels of sensory input even if their purpose is unclear. However, these sensory needs are innate, physiological needs, and it is important to remember that these children must have a certain level of sensory stimuli to be able to attend and engage in higher level learning.

The amount of sensory stimuli a child needs to function at an optimum level is often known as a sensory threshold. Sensory thresholds are unique to the individual and may vary based on other factors. For example, if a child did not get enough sleep the night before, their sensory threshold may be lower than the previous day. As a result, they may not be able to tolerate the extraneous auditory input in the classroom when academic demands are high, such as in math class. On a day when the child receives adequate sleep, the child may not experience any difficulties with too much auditory input and have no problems participating in math. Just as adults may feel stress due to outside factors, such as time constraints or emotional factors, and therefore have less tolerance for sensory stimuli, children experience the same situations. Since sensory processing varies day by day, it is important to get several data points in a variety of situations and environments when assessing sensory processing. This allows the occupational therapist to see patterns and determine if contextual factors contribute to the sensory thresholds.

Examining the sensory threshold of a group or population, rather than the individual, still requires the occupational therapist to look at each individual person as part of the group or population as a whole. However, individuals should only be assessed in how they relate and contribute to the sensory processing of the group or population. In addition, the occupational therapist should consider the group or population as a whole by answering the following questions.

- Is there an overall need for increased stimuli for the group/population?
- Are there times when children are disengaged, have low arousal, and need additional sensory input to alert?
- Are there times when the class appears overwhelmed or at a very high energy level, so much so that they are not able to concentrate on their academic tasks?

When assessing students within the greater classroom population, the occupational therapist can identify groups of students with similar sensory processing patterns and sensory thresholds. This information can be used when establishing groups at the Tier 2 level that have more targeted interventions to meet the specific needs. If there are small groups of students who tend to have a low threshold for sensory input, the occupational therapist can design environmental modifications to decrease sensory stimuli or provide situations that allow for calming sensory inputs. If a group of students tends to have a high threshold for sensory input, the occupational therapist can design highly stimulating activities that provide increased movement, sounds, lights, etc. to help students reach their sensory threshold to engage and complete daily tasks.

When designing interventions to best support students and their sensory thresholds in Tier 1 or Tier 2, a key component that needs to be considered is their alertness to external stimuli throughout their school day. Let us explore how this influences the interventions occupational therapists recommend at population and small group levels after they have collected and interpreted the relevant data.

Impact of Sensory Processing on Alertness Levels

The school day is made up of a series of activities and tasks. Sometimes, these tasks are predictable as part of a student's daily routine. On other days, the tasks and activities vary. In addition to this, each task throughout the day requires a different level of alertness. Some tasks require a low level of alertness, while others require a higher level of alertness, such as those with many physical demands. For example, participation in gym class requires a higher level of alertness than participation in quiet free reading time. As well as tasks that are physically demanding, highly cognitive tasks also require a higher level of alertness to complete. When a student has to concentrate to learn something new, this requires a higher level of alertness than when they are practicing a learned skill on a worksheet.

Some children have trouble changing their alert level between tasks to match the new task, especially if the child has sensory processing differences. For example, a child who increases their alertness level to participate in physical education class may continue to keep their alert level high during quiet study in their next class. On the other hand, if a student has a low alertness level, the attention and concentration needed to complete highly cognitive tasks will be impaired, especially if learning new information is essential to complete a classroom assignment. Highly cognitive tasks create a unique challenge for many students with sensory processing differences, because they are required to remain alert and focused without seeking additional sensory stimuli to keep their engagement level at the optimum. For example, when a child with sensory processing differences is taking a test, their level of alertness must be high to concentrate and demonstrate cognitively what they know. They may require movement to increase their level of alertness. Actively engaging in movement while simultaneously taking a test is often not conducive to the academic testing environment, which can prevent a child from performing at their best level. However, with a few modifications, children can access sensory input to achieve the level of alertness required for the task at hand.

Throughout our day, we all use sensory input to alter our alertness so we can complete our daily tasks to the best of our ability. For instance, many adults choose to exercise and complete their higher cognitive work in the morning as this helps them wake up and organize their schedule, supporting them to perform and meet the demands of their day. For both children and adults, movement is one of the primary sensory systems that we can use to modify our level of alertness. It is important to note, however, that different types of movement can impact our alertness levels in different ways. Children, for example, are often encouraged to jump up and down to increase the amount of movement they receive during the day, which is a type of vertical movement. While this does increase the amount of movement, because it is vertical vestibular movement it also increases their level of alertness, which may not be ideal for a child who needs to complete a test sitting down at a desk. In contrast, linear movement is more calming and tends to help people be more organized. For example, adults take a walk or pace when they experience feelings of stress and anxiety, which changes their alertness level and helps them calm down. Therefore, recommending linear movement, such as taking walks or allowing a child to pace in the classroom, can help change their alertness and increase the amount of movement without overstimulating them.

Visual stimuli are another way many people change their alertness levels consciously or unconsciously. Society is bombarded constantly with fast visual stimuli through visual technology (i.e. phones, tablets, etc.), which greatly impacts and increases a person's level of alertness as it tricks the brain into thinking it is moving. Fast-moving visual stimuli, often seen on phones and tablets, can be interpreted by the brain as alerting vestibular input, thus increasing levels of alertness. Children sometimes crave the increased stimuli from tablets and phones because they do not receive the required amount of movement during the day, and their brain cannot distinguish between fast-moving visual input and vestibular stimuli. In this way, a child may appear to crave visual stimulation when their bodies really need movement to meet their sensory threshold.

Furthermore, auditory stimuli are often overlooked as a contributing factor to a person's level of alertness. In the school setting, children constantly take in and filter auditory stimuli from the environment and other students within the classroom. In addition, much of the information presented in school is presented auditorily, meaning that students must be able to distinguish and filter nonrelevant auditory information, such as the hum of the fan or other students rustling in their desks, and focus on the relevant auditory information presented by the teacher. As a result, auditory stimuli are frequently and easily ignored by individuals who do not display hypo or hyperreactivity to auditory input. A person falling in the expected range of processing auditory stimuli may be unaware of the amount of extraneous noise within an environment because their brain has filtered this stimulus out as irrelevant. Consequently, teachers and caregivers may overlook auditory input as a cause of impacted attention or alertness in class.

The human nervous system is designed to become alert to specific auditory stimuli. As the auditory system is a distance system, it is designed to provide information that is happening away from the body, protecting a person from dangers afar. Hence, a person has time to react and move away from a potentially hazardous situation. Physiologically, the auditory system is designed to be very alarming to the nervous system, causing children with hyperreactivity to auditory input to potentially have heightened levels of alertness throughout the day. Other types of auditory input can be more calming, such as white noise or sound with steady rhythms (for example, 60 beats per minute). Children with auditory sensitivity may hum or make noises to "drown out" the extraneous sounds in their environment. If they make their own noises, they have more control over the auditory stimulus they hear and can dampen the sounds within the environment, which they have no control over.

Finally, there are two types of tactile input to consider when using sensory input to impact level of alertness: deep pressure and light touch. Deep pressure tactile stimulation is calming to the nervous system, which helps the person organize and decrease their alertness even if they are overstimulated by a different sensory input, such as noise. On the other hand, light touch tends to be alerting, especially in the case of unexpected light touch, which often happens in a busy classroom environment full of other children moving about the room. Studies show that hyperreactivity to tactile input can be very disruptive to children during the school day due to the amount of unexpected tactile input from other students, causing overstimulation (Fernández-Andrés et al., 2015). Unexpected light touch can easily increase level of alertness to the point that a child becomes overstimulated rather quickly. To help with this, teachers and school personnel should consider incorporating proprioceptive input into the school day and routine. As a reminder, the proprioceptive system together with the tactile system (somatosensory system) provides information about body position, body awareness, and how the body interacts with the environment. However, it is also an organizing sensory system, meaning the nervous system cannot be hyperresponsive to proprioceptive input. Therefore, incorporating it into tactile input can support children who may have difficulties calming to attend to classroom activities.

To summarize, people react differently to sensory input due to their unique internal sensory processing. Incredibly, a person's reaction to sensory input can change their level of alertness, which impacts their ability to participate and engage at school. By understanding these principles, such as acknowledging the signs of overstimulation and under stimulation, an occupational therapist can incorporate various sensory experiences and inputs throughout the school day that can support students in meeting the demands of school tasks. Before we move forward to how we can address sensory processing needs in the school setting, Table 5.1 can help occupational therapists identify the signs of over and under stimulation, and when calming or alerting sensory inputs should be offered or provided. These signs are general and not specific to a particular student. It is most important to ask the child how their body feels and how sensory input makes their body and mind feel when implementing sensory activities.

Table 5.2 provides some general principles of sensory integration and sensory input on levels of alertness. Again, each person is unique, but these principles tend to be true from a physiological arousal level.

Table 5.1 Signs of Various Levels of Alertness

Signs of Overstimulation	Signs of Under stimulation	Signs of Optimal Level
Increased activity	Lethargic	Engaged in activity
Gaze aversion	Tired	Engaged with others
Moving or pulling away	Difficult to motivate	Facial expressions
Distractibility	Decreased engagement	Able to attend to tasks
Clowning	Head on desk	Able to sequence tasks
Poor ability to separate	Does not engage with	Willing to try new
Difficulties with transitions	others	things
Reluctance to participate in activities		Ease with transitions
Increased whining or expressions of "I can't" or "I don't want to"		
Rage		
Aggressive behaviors		
Explosiveness		

Table 5.2 Generalities in Sensory Input

Tend to be Alerting	Tend to be Calming
Vertical vestibular	Linear vestibular
Light touch	Proprioceptive
Fast moving visual	Deep pressure tactile
Bright colors	Warm/nature colors
Higher auditory tones	Blank walls
	60 beats per minute
	White noise

Addressing Sensory Processing Needs in the School Setting

The role of sensory processing is vital to the success of students in school. Many students can manage their own sensory needs without additional intervention. There are situations built into the school day that allow students to have times of lower sensory stimulation, such as quiet reading time, and times of higher sensory stimulation, such as recess or gym class. Naturally, students go through various levels of alertness throughout the day and are generally able to manage their own sensory needs if provided the opportunity. Therefore, interventions at a Tier 1 level are designed to provide opportunities for all students to meet their sensory needs and remain at the optimal level of alertness for each task during the day. By providing a variety of opportunities during the day to engage in tasks that incorporate movement and heavy work, coupled with times of lower stimulation that incorporate quiet time and lower lighting, many students can have their sensory needs met.

However, some students need additional support or opportunities to ensure their level of alertness is optimal to match the task's demands. Interpreting assessment data allows the occupational therapist to clearly understand how a client processes sensory information regardless of whether the client is a member of a school, classroom, small group, or individual. From this, the occupational therapist will begin to design their interventions using an evidence-based theory.

Choosing a Theory

Occupational therapy practice is based on comprehensive, evidence-based theory that guides intervention. The evidence-based theory provides quality information in the absence of published research evidence and equips the practitioner with a map to outline the therapist's clinical reasoning process. While occupational therapy practitioners must use evidence-informed practice, it is important to know that the profession lacks published evidence for many of the frequently used interventions. However, occupational therapy practice is rooted in evidence that has stood the test of time for over 30 years of implementation. Even when utilizing interventions with high levels of evidence in peer-reviewed publications, occupational therapists must still link the interventions to theory. In the absence of published research, the occupational therapy practitioner can confidently rely on theory to fill in the gaps of evidence and facilitate clinical reasoning and decision-making. Linking evidence-based interventions to theory allows the occupational therapist to adapt evidence and provide individualized interventions that meet the unique needs of each client. Theory guides additional guidance for clinical reasoning and allows the therapist to modify and adapt evidence-based interventions to the needs and response of the client. In other words, theory allows the occupational therapy practitioner to align with evidence-based practice in the absence of published research.

So, how does this look in practice? Evidence-based practice involves using both published evidence and the evidence gathered from working with the specific client in that moment. Then, the therapist uses theory to guide clinical reasoning, performs an evidence-based intervention while adapting it to the setting and needs of the client, and ultimately evaluates the effectiveness of the intervention based on the client's response. After this, the therapist uses this evidence to modify or implement the intervention based on the client's reaction. This constant evaluation of the client's performance is a method of evidence-based practice and is essential to the success of occupational therapy practice.

In Ayres Sensory Integration®, the process of evaluating intervention effectiveness based on the client's response is known as data-driven decision-making (DDDM). Data-driven decision-making is a step-by-step process that guides a therapist in the implementation of sensory interventions to ensure maximum effectiveness with a particular client, whether that client be a population, group, or individual (Schaaf & Mailloux, 2015). It is outlined in specifics in the *Clinician's Guide for Implementing Ayres Sensory Integration®: Promoting Participation for Children with Autism* by Schaaf and Mailloux (2015). The process consists of eight steps that guide the therapist in the evaluation, analysis, treatment planning, and monitoring of outcomes. It is part of the manualized intervention process for the implementation of ASI, but can be applied to all areas of occupational therapy. Table 5.3 is an overview of each step of the DDDM process and how they may be modified to apply to the Tier 1 and Tier 2 levels of intervention. Next, we will turn to different evidence-based theories occupational therapists can choose from when designing interventions within these tiers.

Person-Environment-Occupation

The Person-Environment-Occupation, or PEO, theory was developed by Law and colleagues (1996) and is an excellent theoretical framework to utilize when applying interventions at Tier 1 and Tier 2 levels. The PEO model functions

Table 5.3 Modifying DDDM Steps to apply to Tier 1 and Tier 2

Step of DDDM	Description	Modification to Tier 1 and Tier 2 and Application
Step one	Identify strengths and participation challenges	This step at a Tier 1/Tier 2 level involves getting to know the teacher, classroom, district, and structure of how students interact within this system
Step two	Describe the current level and factors affecting participation	Synthesize information on what supports participation and what may hinder participation; focus on the environment and context
Step three	Conduct the assessment	Assessment/evaluation phase; under Tier 1/Tier 2 this is frequently done through interviews, observation, and questionnaires
Step four	Develop and set goals	Goals should focus on increasing participation; they may also focus on training staff outcomes (which are discussed below)
Step five	Identify outcome measures	The district or school often provides outcome measures, however, occupational therapists should have a systematic way of gathering and tracking outcomes (this will be discussed in more detail in the next chapter)
Step six	Generate hypothesis	The hypothesis should use data to link proximal sensory outcomes to distal participation difficulties
Step seven	Conduct the intervention	The intervention should be targeted toward the hypothesis to address proximal outcomes moving to distal outcomes
Step eight	Measure outcomes and monitor progress	Interventions are modified, continued, or discontinued based on data from their implementation and gathered from progress monitoring (this will be discussed further in the next chapter)

(Mailloux and Schaaf, 2015)

under the assumption that the person and environment interact, with the outcome being occupational performance. The better the fit between the person and environment, the better the occupational performance. Dysfunction can occur when there is a poor fit between the person and the environment. This may be when the person's abilities or expectations differ from what is produced in the environment, or when the environmental demands are higher or lower than what the person can produce. The goal of intervention under this model is to increase the fit between the person and environment, and in turn to increase occupational performance.

The first intervention method under this theory is to intervene in the environment. Therefore, when using this theory to address sensory processing, the occupational therapist should first look to modify the environment to increase the fit between the person and the environment. In the case of MTSS Tier 1 and Tier 2, the person is the population of the school or classroom, or the (small) group of students (Tier 2). The environment can be easily manipulated by changing aspects of the physical and sensory environment, routines of the client, or the persons within the environment. In this chapter, the PEO theory will be utilized the most in guiding and identifying interventions under MTSS at the Tier 1 and Tier 2 levels.

Ayres Sensory Integration®

Ayre Sensory Integration® (ASI) was developed by A. Jean Ayres and is the original theory and frame of reference for the foundation of all sensory interventions in occupational therapy (1979). Since the inception of the theory, many other aspects of sensory interventions have been included to accompany the original theory and intervention of sensory integration. Under ASI, key principles need to be followed during the intervention to maintain its fidelity (Parham et al., 2011). The overarching focus of ASI is on the therapist providing opportunities for enhanced sensory experiences to facilitate an adaptive response. The person must initiate the activity for the adaptive response, and there has to be active participation of the person in the intervention (Bundy & Lane, 2020). The framework focuses on modifying, or remediating, sensory processing differences using a strength-based approach toward utilizing stronger sensory systems to help integrate systems that may be having difficulty. The goal of ASI is to improve participation and help a child internalize adaptive processes so they can apply them throughout their day to participate in daily tasks.

This theory was originally designed to be individualized and therefore is most ideal to utilize at the Tier 3 level. That being said, many principles from ASI can be applied to interventions presented in the Tier 1 and Tier 2 levels. In fact, although sensory-based interventions are not considered ASI, they were developed from Ayres's original theory of sensory integration and processing. Sensory-based interventions, sensory techniques, and ASI all fall under the broader category of sensory interventions.

It is crucial for occupational therapy practitioners to be able to distinguish sensory interventions from ASI to maintain fidelity and understanding of ASI by those who are not occupational therapists. Additionally, they must also understand the connection between sensory interventions and the original ASI theory, and must have the ability to readily explain the differences between the intervention of ASI and other sensory interventions. Sensory interventions, namely sensory-based interventions or sensory techniques, are often performed by an adult to a child (Case-Smith et al., 2015), or the environment is set up so that the child can access specific sensory input and apply the input themselves. Unlike ASI, with sensory-based interventions there is no need for active participation of the child when applying the sensory-based interventions. That also means that the goal of sensory interventions is not to make lasting changes in how the nervous system processes sensory information. Instead, the goal is to change the child's level of alertness to better match the demands of the task and environment (Case-Smith et al., 2015). Therefore, when utilizing sensory-based interventions, the occupational therapist seeks to better match the client's physiological arousal level to the task, which is similar to the PEO model.

The goals of the school-based occupational therapist are to act as a related service to help students access and fully participate in the activities and learning of the school setting. Some districts may interpret this to define the role of occupational therapy according to a remediation model, which would warrant ASI being implemented. Other districts function more so under the idea that occupational therapists are there to help facilitate and support access to curriculum and other school activities. Therefore, the model utilized under Tier 1 and Tier 2 would be applied to Tier 3, just under a more individualized and intensified method. However, recent research has shown positive effects of utilizing ASI in the school setting when also working with teachers to implement strategies in the classroom. Improvements in participation and functional regulation were shown in students who received ASI for only 15 weeks (approximately one semester) in the school setting (Whiting et al., 2023), showing how the principles of ASI can be implemented at Tier 1 and 2 levels.

Ecology of Human Performance

The Ecology of Human Performance (EHP) was developed by Dunn and colleagues (1994) and provides another optional framework for applying sensory interventions at the Tier 1 and Tier 2 levels. The framework focuses on the relationship between the person, context, tasks, and performance. However, the interaction of the person and environment is key to this framework. It considers the cognitive, psychosocial, and sensorimotor skills of the person that exist within a given context, and it believes that the environment can either support or hinder performance. Interventions in EHP may function under a few methods, including establishing or restoring skills and abilities of the person; altering the environment or context; adapting the task, task demands, or environment; preventing maladaptation or poor fit of the person and context; and creating opportunities for improved performance within contexts.

Under this framework, occupational therapy is viewed as most effective when it occurs within the natural context and flow of life, making it an excellent theory to guide school-based practice. As interventions should be implemented in the least restrictive environment, sensory interventions applied under this theory are ideal when provided at Tier 1 and Tier 2 levels. The interventions are designed to take place in the natural context, which aligns with IDEA and the least restrictive environment (LRE) to provide intervention services in the child's classroom and within their regular schedule whenever possible. The EHP theory promotes the implementation of occupational therapy interventions within the "real life" setting of the child.

Next, the intervention discusses the importance of altering the environment and context so that the context can facilitate rather than hinder a person's performance. Occupational therapists are experts in task analysis, so they can easily provide modifications and adaptations to ensure the child succeeds in school-related activities and retains their access to the required learning activities. As well as adaptation being a central focus of EHP, it is also vital under IDEA. The occupational therapist can work with the IEP team to design modifications and accommodations to change tasks and environmental demands to help create an environment more conducive to the success of the child.

Finally, this framework works well in the school setting because it also focuses on prevention. The goal of early intervening services is to prevent the need for more intensified and individualized services that may stop a child from having full access to the LRE. The EHP theory can justify integrating interventions at lower-tier levels before issues arise in the hopes of preventing future difficulties for students. The occupational therapist can anticipate potential difficulties students at the population, group, and individual levels may encounter and design interventions at Tier 1 and Tier 2 levels to prevent these difficulties from even occurring in the first place. This can help ensure the success of all students within the context of the LRE.

Unlike the PEO model, EHP provides the first phase of intervention with the person, whereas the PEO model first intervenes at the environment, followed by the person. Since Tier 1 and Tier 2 interventions should focus more on the environment, the PEO theoretical model is chosen for the interventions in this chapter. The goal is first to provide interventions targeting the environment to increase the fit between the person (in this case, the population or group) and the environment, thus improving occupational performance. If the intervention targeting the environment is successful, there is no need for intervention targeted at the person.

Once an occupational therapy practitioner has chosen an evidence-based theory, it is essential they develop goals to drive their interventions. This is so they can monitor whether they are positively helping the sensory processing needs of their client, adapting their interventions as required to best support their students. We will now explore how this can be done effectively and qualitatively.

Developing Goals

It cannot be understated how essential it is for the occupational therapist to write high-quality goals when implementing interventions in a school setting. This is because well-written goals allow the therapists and other school personnel to track progress, stay focused, and have a clear picture of the intervention's effectiveness. But, how is this achieved?

During the goal-setting process, it is important to begin by defining exactly who the client is. The school-based occupational therapist needs to remember that goals written for Tier 1 and Tier 2 interventions are not targeted toward one individual, instead the client consists of a population or group. When working at a Tier 1 level, the client may be the entire school, everyone who attends music class, or a specific classroom (i.e. Ms. Jones's second grade class). In contrast, as Tier 2 is working with students who have already been identified as having some additional needs, this information can be used to define the client in the goal. For example, a client may be described as "A group of five students from Ms. Jones's second grade classroom that have sensory-seeking tendencies."

After defining the client in the goal, the intent of the intervention should be provided and defined. At the population level (Tier 1), the goal may be for students to remain engaged in seated desk work for the duration of the oral reading period. The specifics of the goal will be what is identified in the assessment process, such as the number of prompts needed for students to remain seated, or the amount of time the students should remain seated.

The next step is to provide a method of measuring progress (which will be explored in depth in Chapter 6). This should be a simple method so that teachers and other school personnel can easily track and provide data for the goal. When occupational therapists write goals, they need to remember how data will be collected so that progress and data can be gathered easily and quickly. Teachers and school personnel are busy with many things and must collect a lot of data throughout the day. Easy tracking methods, such as check marks or tally marks, can help ensure consistent data collection compliance.

Finally, the goal should include a timeline and criteria to determine if the goal has been met. Since many districts do progress monitoring every four weeks, percentages are a nice way to monitor progress and allow for the fluctuation of performance that naturally occurs. Using graphs to plot data can also help reveal trends, in addition to percentages. Percentages and averages allow for many data points to be analyzed succinctly and provide usable information to determine the success of interventions.

You can see an example of goal setting in Box 5.1. In this scenario, the goal would have been set and defined after an assessment had taken place.

BOX 5.1   EXAMPLE OF GOAL SETTING

Area of concern: The teacher reported that students move around the room, are loud, and have difficulty paying attention during oral reading time. As a result, they are struggling to retain the information from the reading to summarize and answer questions.

Assessment results: Several students had an increased need for movement (hyporeactivity to vestibular) and, therefore, had difficulties sitting for long periods. The classroom also had a lot of extraneous noises from the lights, fans, and students moving around.

Goal: Students will remain seated during the duration of oral reading time (approximately 20 minutes) with no more than one verbal prompt from the teacher or the teacher assistant.

Intervention:

*   Provide opportunities for students to use alternative seating, such as rocking chairs and therapy balls.
*   Provide an area of the classroom where students can quietly pace while listening to the story.
*   Turn off appliances that may be causing excessive noise.
*   Dim the lights in one area of the room.
*   Provide a visual orientation to allow students to follow along with the story, which will assist with visual focus and attention.

Progress monitoring and tracking: Note the duration of reading time and the number of prompts provided to the students for attention during that time.

In contrast to students receiving therapy services under Tier 3, goals for Tier 1 and Tier 2 interventions may be overlooked as they are often not required to be established and monitored. However, it is still important to ensure goals are established and are measurable to determine effectiveness of the interventions provided and to clearly establish the desired outcome of the intervention.

Below are some examples of goals you may write for Tier 1 and Tier 2.

Tier 1 Goals

*   Students will recognize physical signs of different emotions and independently choose a sensory activity to regulate to perform classroom activities.
*   Students will learn and use basic self-regulation sensory strategies when feeling overwhelmed.

- Students will follow established classroom routines and understand expectations for behavior using sensory tools and supports as needed to follow classroom routines and behavior expectations.
- When provided prompts, students will apply self-regulation sensory strategies during academic tasks to maintain the level of alertness needed to complete the task.

Tier 2 Goals

- Students will create and implement a personalized sensory coping plan for specific triggers or challenging situations.
- Students will regularly self-monitor and reflect on their behavioral and emotional responses, implementing sensory strategies when needed to demonstrate expected behaviors and emotions.
- Students will develop effective social problem-solving skills to navigate peer interactions and conflicts, using sensory strategies as needed to calm during social situations.
- Students will develop effective problem-solving skills and utilize sensory strategies to navigate peer interactions and academic routines when they feel overwhelmed or frustrated.

Now, let us apply this practically to how an occupational therapist would design and implement interventions in the school setting.

How to Design Interventions

When designing interventions to address sensory processing needs at the Tier 1 and Tier 2 levels, the occupational therapist should first choose a theoretical basis for the occupational therapy process. As mentioned, this chapter will primarily utilize the PEO theory to design and implement interventions. With this in mind, we will explore different interventions we can implement to modify the environment to help students with sensory processing needs and improve their occupational performance.

Modifying the Environment

Occupational therapy defines context as being composed of environmental and personal factors. Environmental factors include a person's physical, social, and attitudinal surroundings, whereas other considerations of the environment include the natural and human-made environment, products, technology, support, relationships, attitudes, services, systems, and policies (AOTA, 2020).

SENSORY ENVIRONMENT

The sensory environment can be modified or changed to create a better physical environment for students to learn and function in based on their sensory processing. Items within the environment can be placed in or removed from the environment to encourage engagement in sensory activities. Table 5.4 provides examples of sensory related environmental modifications. We will explore the sensory environment in detail below.

VISUAL ENVIRONMENT

The visual environment is easily modified and can generate a more conducive learning environment. It can also be designed to encourage focused visual attention on desired visual stimuli, such as the board or the teacher, supporting students who need more sensory input to be engaged. On the other hand, by modifying the visual environment to be less stimulating, this can help students who are distracted by too much visual input or those who have difficulty filtering to focus on specified visual input. Below are a few examples of ways you can modify the environment to help make the learning space calmer for students who are hyperreactive to visual input, and ways to make the classroom more engaging for students who are hyporeactive to visual input.

Environmental modifications for students that are **hyperreactive** to visual input:

- decrease items on the walls
- use natural colors, such as tans, light greens, blues,
- keep desk and table spaces clear
- arrange furniture into clearly defined spaces
- lower the lighting by using light covers or natural light
- create spaces in corners of rooms that provide a visual boundary
- allow students to wear hats and sunglasses to block lights
- draw the shades.

Environmental modifications for students that are **hyporeactive** to visual input:

- feature bright colors and patterns
- increase lighting
- provide visually stimulating items such as lava lamps, bubble timers, spinning objects, etc.
- provide visual schedules and visual handouts
- highlight areas of importance on worksheets or information presented on the board
- increase lighting in areas that need additional visual attention.

Table 5.4 Sensory-Based Interventions and Environmental Modifications

Sensory System	Sensory-Based Intervention/Environmental Modification
Visual	• Light covers • Lamps instead of overhead lights • Natural lighting • Closing the shades • Dimming lights or turning lights off • Bubble lamps • Wearing sunglasses • Wearing hats • Sensory calm-down jars • Decreasing items on walls and desks • Darker area of the room, such as a tent • Color code schedules • Visual schedules • Access to visual tools (kaleidoscopes, spinning toys, bubble timers, etc.
Auditory	• Headphones • Ear plugs • Headbands over ears • Listening to music in headphones • Calming music (classical or 60 beats per minute) • Metronomes • Quiet corner
Tactile	• Variety of weighted items (lap pads, blankets, neck weights, ankle weights, etc.) • Velcro under the desk • Variety of fidgets • Sensory tables/tubs with various media (i.e. beans, rice, shaving cream, slime, etc.) • Defined areas for sitting and standing in line to prevent unexpected touch, such as taped squares on the floor or mats to sit on
Olfactory	• A scent-free area of the classroom • Open windows • Smelling station with various scented oils • Calming scents such as lavender using diffusers or candles
Vestibular	• Flexible seating options (i.e. rocking chairs, T-stools, balls, move-n-sit cushions, etc.) • Opportunities to stand at the desk instead of sit • Jump and touch station • Head shakes • Allow for free movement in the classroom
Proprioceptive	• Tie resistance bands to chair legs so students can push their feet on it • Chair push-ups • Kinesthetic learning opportunities • Oral input (chewies, straws, resistive water bottles, etc.) • Classroom cleaning activities (putting books away, cleaning the board, cleaning desks, etc.)

Some general visual sensory environmental modifications that the occupational therapy practitioner can suggest to classroom teachers include the following.

- Decreasing clutter in the classroom and on the walls helps students know where to focus visual attention and creates a calmer environment overall.
- Making sure to keep desk and table areas clean and organized, decreasing the amount of furniture in the room, and having few things on the walls will create a calmer space.

For students in Tier 2 who have more identified needs, small group spaces should be created that are less cluttered. In addition, providing visual supports, such as visual schedules, can help students stay focused and provide an environmental cue toward independence.

AUDITORY ENVIRONMENT

There are many extraneous noises in the classroom and school environment. Some can be controlled, while others may be out of the direct control of the teacher or administration. Much of the information presented during instructional time is auditory. Therefore, it is important to help students focus their auditory attention on the learning instruction and decrease extraneous noises when possible.

Environmental modifications for students that are **hyperreactive** to auditory input:

- place noise-dampening materials on the walls/floors
- place balls on the bottoms of chairs
- allow students to put up their hoods or wear headbands
- allow earplugs/headphones
- play calming background music at 60 beats per minute.

Environmental modifications for students that are **hyporeactive** to auditory input:

- encourage students to sit near the area where the teacher is talking
- listen to music on headphones
- provide auditory feedback during reading time.

BOX 5.2   A NOTE ON HEADPHONES

Noise-canceling headphones have become increasingly popular as a sensory-based strategy for individuals with auditory sensitivities. While these can be effective for short-term and incidental situations, noise-canceling headphones should not be used excessively. Noise-canceling headphones can be effective for certain situations, such as loud assemblies, or when there is a need for a high level of attention, such as during a test. However, overuse of headphones does not promote adaptation and can prevent students from becoming more engaged in classroom activities. Noise-canceling headphones may not allow students to fully engage in the learning and social processes in the school environment. In fact, one study by Ikuta and colleagues (2016) examined the use of earmuffs, noise-canceling headphones, and no ear covering to see which was the most effective in addressing goals related to auditory sensitivities. The noise-canceling headphones were not found to result in statistically significant changes, while the earmuff wearing did result in statistically significant changes. Although this is only one study, it indicates that decreasing auditory stimuli, rather than entirely blocking auditory stimuli, may be more effective for students with auditory sensitivities. Proper assessment will allow the occupational therapist to design times when headphones should be available for use in a Tier 1 model, and also more specific times for group interventions at the Tier 2 level. The occupational therapist can help design a schedule for when headphones may be warranted for students with auditory sensitivities.

TACTILE ENVIRONMENT

As mentioned before, unexpected tactile touch is common in a busy school environment, but it can be extremely disruptive, especially to students who have hyperreactivity to tactile input. Therefore, it is important to consider how to space students in structured and unstructured times of the day to decrease the chances of unexpected tactile input. For example, school personnel could increase the space between desks, assign specific spaces for each student during floor time, and even map out distance between students when lining up, such as standing on a tile on the floor with one tile between each student.

Furthermore, providing opportunities for deep pressure tactile input throughout the day and at different places in the classroom can allow students to regulate their nervous systems with tactile input. Students can provide deep pressure tactile to themselves with arm and leg squeezes, commercial massagers (note that these often also provide vibration, which is often simulating to the vestibular system), and weighted items. Other examples are included below.

Methods to increase tactile input in the classroom:

- commercial fidgets
- other fidgets (for example, paperclips)

- stress balls
- Velcro on bottom of desk
- fabric swatches
- blankets and pillows in quiet areas or reading corners
- fabrics on chairs
- different types of carpeting to sit on during circle time.

BOX 5.3   A NOTE ON WEIGHTED ITEMS

Weighted items can provide a great opportunity for calming input and can be made available for all students under Tier 1. Many commercially available items are weighted, including lap pads, neck wraps, blankets, vests, and animals. However, these weighted items can also be made, and it is important to have various weights of items available for children of different sizes. For Tier 2, providing weighted items for the group of students during times when they need to perform seated activities is a way to make the intervention more targeted toward the needs of a specific group.

Figure 5.1 provides some examples of weighted items including cuff weights, weighted vests, and weighted blankets. Figure 5.2 shows an example of a weighted lap pad that a child can place on their lap during seated activities.

BOX 5.4   HOW TO MAKE A WEIGHTED LAP PAD

An easy way to make a weighted lap pad is to use a pillowcase. Cut the pillowcase in half and fill it with bean bag pellets. Sew the end together and it is ready for use.

We have now explored varying ways occupational therapists can modify the environment to support the sensory processing of the students, promoting a universal design for learning. In this next section, we will define and review different cognitive-based regulation programs to help children perform their best in the school environment. At the end of this chapter, we will share examples of sensory supports that can be implemented at these different tiers.

Sensory Supports at the Tier 1 and Tier 2 Level

Sensory environmental modifications are key when implementing a sensory program at a Tier 1 level. However, designing sensory activities that meet the needs of

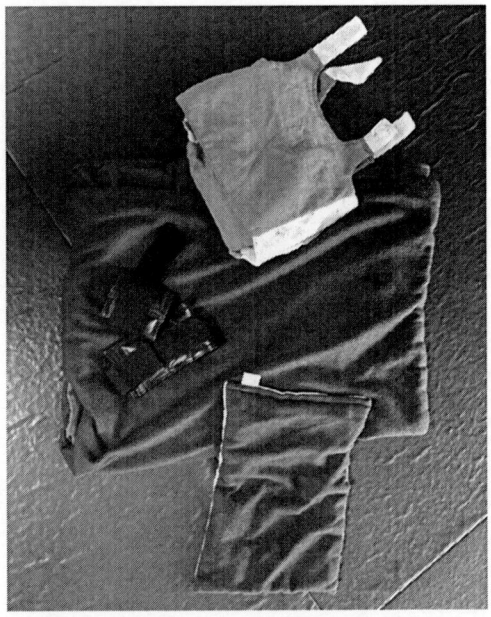

Figure 5.1 Various weighted items. Image by author.

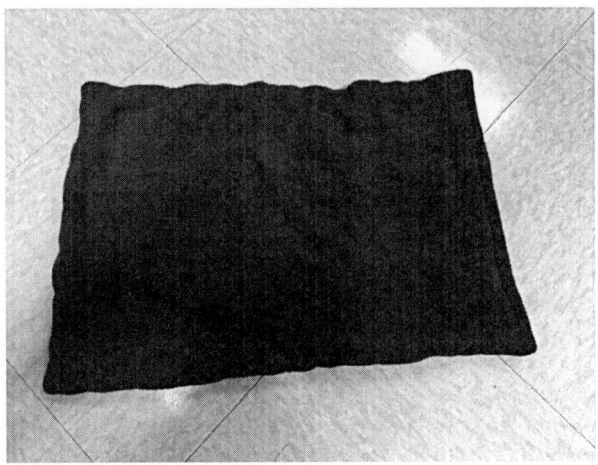

Figure 5.2 Weighted lap pad. Image by author.

the classroom is also a key component of sensory interventions implemented at an MTSS Tier 1 level. When designing sensory supports for implementation at a Tier 2 level, the occupational therapist can be more intentional on grouping students together that have similar sensory needs. This allows the occupational therapy practitioner to design direct sensory interventions to meet the specific needs of the group. For example, the occupational therapist may identify a group of four students that require increased vestibular input and design a movement-based sensory group time each morning and afternoon to help build additional vestibular input into the daily routine. As a Tier 2 intervention, the goal would be to increase the attention and on-task behavior of the students, and the small group sensory time would be implemented with the already established Tier 1 interventions.

Sensory activities can be performed in isolation, with one sensory input provided at a time or in a sequence of sensory activities. When designing interventions that focus on a sequence of activities, it is best to use a calming strategy as the final activity. Typically, proprioceptive or deep-pressure tactile activities should be the final activity before returning to classroom activities.

Next, we will explore a list of sensory activities that can be used to design school-wide, classroom, or small group sensory activities to embed within the school day. Since some children have difficulties processing sensory information, this may cause them to have behavior difficulties, trouble with transitions, difficulties with learning and attention, or difficulties with motor skills. Using the list below, the occupational therapy practitioner can design opportunities for sensory input throughout the day and can help organize the nervous system to function better in the school environment. Each sensory system will be addressed with a list of activities along with their main purpose. These activities can be used to design a program for groups of students with sensory processing needs.

Vestibular Activities

As a reminder, the vestibular system is our movement system. Vestibular input has a direct impact on our arousal levels and attention. Some vestibular input is organizing and some is alerting. Organizing activities should be used when students attend and focus on seated work and when they need to decrease their level of arousal to focus on academics, such as after lunch. In addition, many students do not receive the necessary amount of vestibular input needed during the day. Therefore, building in additional vestibular opportunities throughout the day is key to maintaining attention and focus.

ORGANIZING ACTIVITIES

Organizing activities include the following:

- Swinging
- Taking a walk

- Swaying in a hammock
- Rocking in a rocking chair
- Rhythmic rolling on a large therapy ball
- Scooter board
- Lying on your back over a large ball with your feet on the ground.

Provide movement opportunities throughout the day to help students reach their movement needs, such as:

- Jumping on a trampoline
- Jumping 10–20 times to touch the upper threshold of the door or an identified target on the wall
- Sitting and spinning in an office chair
- Bouncing on a large therapy ball
- Dancing
- Marching
- Twirling
- Jumping rope
- Imitating head positions
- Shaking and stretching your body
- Passing a ball overhead and through the legs
- Somersaults.

Although many of these movement opportunities are alerting, which is necessary for some students to engage and organize, some students may have difficulty calming themselves after alerting vestibular input. Therefore, following these vestibular activities with proprioceptive activities or deep-pressure tactile can help calm the nervous system.

Proprioceptive Activities

Proprioception has its receptors in our muscles and joints and is responsible for body awareness. It is the one sensory system that cannot display a hyperreactivity, and therefore it is always designed for organizing. Proprioceptive activities should be performed either in conjunction with vestibular activities or immediately after vestibular activities whenever possible. Providing opportunities for pushing, pulling, climbing, and heavy work multiple times throughout the school day will help students stay regulated and organized to perform school-related tasks. Implementing several heavy work proprioceptive activities throughout the day will also help students stay organized all day. By providing opportunities for squeezing and pinching, students are able to increase proprioceptive input while still attending to and participating in seated desk work or other seated activities, such as circle time. Finally, oral input is the most organizing type of proprioceptive input and should be used when students need additional calming input. It is also something students can participate in while still performing academic tasks.

PUSHING/PULLING/CLIMBING

- Pushing a toy shopping cart filled with heavy items (i.e. books).
- Pushing a laundry basket full of wet or dry laundry.
- Pulling a wagon.
- Pushing another child on a riding toy.
- Vacuuming.
- Tug of war.
- Monkey bars.
- Rock walls.
- Climbing on playground equipment.
- Climbing a rope or suspended ladder.

HEAVY WORK

- Animal walks.
- Wheelbarrow walking.
- Wall and chair push-ups.
- Crawling games or maintaining a crawling position for 1–2 minutes.
- Carrying heavy objects (dishes to help set the table, books, backpack with books, laundry basket, etc.).
- Scrubbing the floor.
- Commando crawl.
- Moving furniture.
- Wearing weighted items (backpack with books, weighted vest, lap pad, etc.)
- Lying on tummy over pillow/towel bolster to weight bear on arms.
- Cleaning boards, windows, tables.
- Helping with vacuuming and sweeping.
- Pressing hands together.
- Joint compressions.

SQUEEZING/PINCHING

- Cutting playdough with scissors and hiding objects in it for the child to find.
- Therapy putty.
- Rolling pin.
- Hole punch.
- Sidewalk chalk.

- Squeezing clothespins.
- Stress balls and other fidget toys.

ORAL INPUT

The mouth is one of the most sensitive areas of the body. Input to the mouth can be very calming and organizing. The following are oral input that can be provided throughout the school day.

- Chewy foods (beef jerky, gummies, Twizzlers, bagels, soft pretzels, large hard pretzels, raisins, granola bars, gum).
- Chewing gum.
- Resistive sucking (use straws to drink liquids, yogurt, milkshakes, pudding).
- Chewy tools.
- Blow toys (pin wheel, bubbles, balloons, etc.)
- Have students imitate funny faces with their mouth/tongue.

Tactile Activities

The tactile system is comprised of our largest sensory organ, the skin. Therefore, we take in a lot of information through our tactile sense. Some students have difficulty with tactile discrimination and tactile hyperactivity, causing them to need additional tactile activities. Deep pressure is calming to the nervous system and can be used to promote a decrease in level of alertness. The activities listed below should be used whenever students need to organize or calm. They are excellent for situations where students may experience anxiety. Tactile opportunities should be plentiful in the classrooms for preschool and lower elementary students as their tactile systems continue to develop.

DEEP PRESSURE (CALMING)

- Arm and leg squeezes.
- Back massages.
- Towel rubdowns with deep pressure after bath or swimming.
- Pillow squishes.
- Wrapping in a heavy blanket with head out and press pillow on top of student's body.
- Rolling a large ball over the student's back.
- Lotion massages.
- Wearing tight-fitting clothing (compression clothing).
- Bear hugs.
- Towel and blanket snuggles.

OTHER TACTILE ACTIVITIES

- Playing in a variety of textures (sand, water, play-do, silly putty, cookie dough, oatmeal, finger paints, shaving cream, rice beans, brushes, creams).
- Hiding objects in textures and have students use their hands to search for objects.
- Fidget toys.
- Rubbing lotion or powder on the student while they identify body parts.
- Painting body parts with a clean paintbrush.
- Water play.
- Soap paint.
- Finger painting with paints, pudding, applesauce, and frosting.
- Playing in ball pits.
- Snow angels on carpet.
- Log rolling over various fabrics and down a grassy hill.
- Playing dress-up with costumes made of various fabrics.

SENSORY BINS

Fill bins with the following items.

- Dry rice, beans, or pasta,
- Sand.
- Shredded paper.
- Soapy water.
- Shaving cream.

FIDGETS

Provide a variety of options for fidgets for students to use throughout the day as needed.

- Hand-held back massager.
- Stress balls.
- Rubber bands or hair elastics/scrunchies.
- Keyrings.
- Watch bands with Velcro closures.
- Bracelets.
- Stretch toys.
- Koosh ball.
- Pipe cleaners.
- Putty.
- Spinning toys.
- Fans.
- Pinwheels.

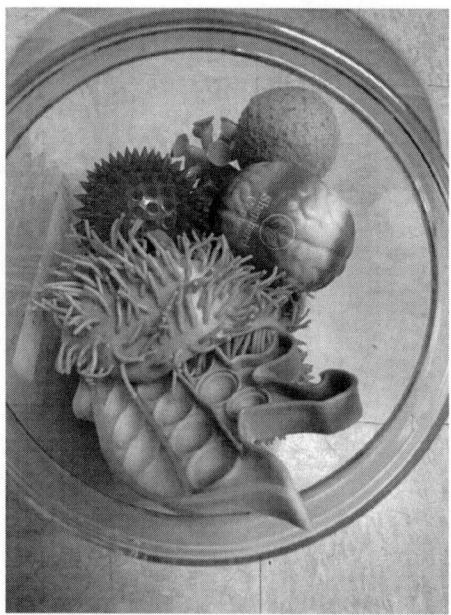

Figure 5.3 Variety of fidgets. Image by author.

Auditory/Visual

Auditory input can be calming or disruptive. Allowing students to access different sounds on their own personal listening devices can provide calming input to students who need auditory input to calm without disrupting other students. Some auditory input, such as white noise or music/metronomes at 60 beats per minute can promote an organizing atmosphere.

AUDITORY

- Personal music on headphones.
- Noise-canceling headphones.
- Classroom music at 60 beats per minute.
- White noise.
- Ear plugs.

Visual input can provide a way for students to organize and focus visual information. At times students may need to focus on visual stimuli, such as a bubble timer, in order to decrease visual distractions from the environment.

VISUAL

- Bubble timers.
- Spinning toys.
- Kaleidoscopes.
- Flashlight tags.
- Light tables.
- Sensory bottles.
- Marble mazes.

Figure 5.4 provides a sample sensory program for a first grade classroom.

Support for Free Play in the School Setting

Free play is essential for physical, social, emotional, and mental well-being. It supports all areas of development, including cognitive, emotional, physical, and sensory. Incorporating free play into the regular school day routine is one of the most effective ways to ensure children can meet their sensory needs. Free play differs from structured play in that children can engage in any activity they choose. Remember, sensory processing needs are physiological needs. That means that the body will seek to meet that need. Like with hunger, thirst, or sleep, a child will work to ensure that need is satisfied before worrying about other things like schoolwork, attending to the teacher, and engaging with others. When children are allowed the opportunity to engage in free play regularly, they are allowed to meet their sensory needs in the best way their body requires. When free play is withheld or does not occur as frequently as needed, the child may engage in other sensory seeking behaviors throughout the day.

Free play is unstructured and voluntary. The child always initiates it, although the environment can provide play opportunities. For example, equipment sets the stage for play opportunities when children play on a playground. One crucial aspect of free play regarding sensory needs is that free play allows a child opportunities to explore different activities. Through exploration, the child can determine if the activity meets their sensory needs and if they can reach their sensory threshold. It helps the child understand what activities make their mind and body feel differently and how to regulate their sensory systems through unstructured play. Children gain confidence in their understanding of their bodies and needs, which can lead to increased autonomy in regulating sensory systems and engaging in activities that help to regulate their nervous system while remaining on task and participating in classroom routines.

Recess is one of the most critical aspects of the school day. It provides the opportunity for children to engage in free play, which supports all of the learning and behavior goals that teachers try to promote in the classroom setting. Free gross motor play facilitates cognitive development, emotional development,

Sensory Program

Classroom/Group: _____Ms. Smith's First Grade Class_____

When to Implement (Time of Day or Activity): _____Upon Arrival_____
How Long to Implement: _____10 minutes_____

Sensory System	Activity Choices	Goal
Vestibular	Jumping jacks	Alerting movement
Tactile	Arm squeezes	Calming input
Proprioception	Crab walk to front of room and back to desk	Heavy work organizing input

When to Implement (Time of Day or Activity): _____After Lunch_____
How Long to Implement: _____5 minutes_____

Sensory System	Activity Choices	Goal
Vestibular	n/a	Students should have had movement at lunch and need organizing input
Proprioception	10 wall push ups	Heavy work organizing input
Tactile	Give self three bear hugs	Calming input

When to Implement (Time of Day or Activity): _____Before small group reading time_____
How Long to Implement: _____15 minutes_____

Sensory System	Activity Choices	Goal
Vestibular	Infinity walk around the classroom with follow the leader	Increase movement that is organizing
Proprioception	Animal walk Simon says	Increase heavy work for organizing input

Comments:

Figure 5.4 Sample sensory program. Image by author.

and attention and problem-solving. Children have many opportunities to participate in gross motor activities during recess. These activities promote sensory integration and processing and help ensure sensory development is facilitated and sensory needs are met. Playgrounds have many vestibular opportunities, including swings and spinning equipment. In addition, children can participate in vestibular activities, such as running and jumping, which promote regulation, body awareness, spatial orientation, balance, and coordination. Further, much of the playground equipment is set up to encourage proprioceptive input, such as climbing, hanging, pushing, and pulling. Equipment such as monkey bars and climbing structures allow children to have increased input to muscles and joints to support body awareness, overall organization, and motor planning. The playground also has many tactile opportunities, including different textures and temperatures. In addition, children may experience various touch from others on the playground. While unexpected touch may be disruptive in the classroom, when provided with increased organizing sensory input while experiencing unexpected touch, the nervous system is better able to regulate and not over respond. Beyond vestibular, proprioceptive, and tactile input, children experience auditory and visual stimulation on the playground and must integrate and organize that information while playing. Since the child initiates free play, the child is free to start and stop any activity as they please. As a result, they learn to regulate and integrate sensory information that may overwhelm them in another setting where they do not have control.

Since recess is one of the most important and simple ways to meet the needs of all children, including those with and without sensory processing differences, recess should not be used as a reward, nor should withholding recess be used as a punishment. Since sensory needs are physiological, withholding the opportunity to engage in these free play activities where sensory needs can be met would be equivalent to withholding food from a child. Children should be allowed to participate in recess at least twice a day for 30–45 minutes each session.

Teachers and occupational therapists must advocate with parents and school administrators for additional free play recess time. Educating parents on the importance of allowing children to engage in free play during the morning before school is also important to the success of the school day. Advocating for safe play areas before school starts allows students to be dropped off early and engage in free play in a secure environment. In addition, the occupational therapist should play a vital role in promoting and advocating for recess time in the school setting. The occupational therapist is an expert in play and sensory development and can teach school administrators the importance of free play. Preschool and school-age students should have a minimum of one to three hours of free daily active play (CDC Physical Activity Basics, 2024; Koepp et al., 2022). Therefore, encouraging parents to provide opportunities for free play before and after school is important.

In addition, promoting free play time through recess is an excellent way to incorporate sensory integration opportunities for the entire school at the Tier 1 level. By utilizing recess as a Tier 1 intervention, occupational therapy practitioners can gather the required data and demonstrate the effectiveness of free play to promote its implementation school- and district-wide. To achieve this, occupational therapists should gain administrative support for implementing increased recess time as a Tier 1 intervention. They should then choose targeted behaviors to monitor, take baseline data, and then monitor the progress of these goals. Some behaviors to consider are referrals to the principal's office, safety-related goals, attendance, and anti-bullying/promoting kindness goals through social and emotional curriculums.

Here are some sample goal areas that may be supported by increased recess time in social and emotional learning.

- Reduce incidents of bullying and foster a positive school climate.
- Reduce the number of behavioral referrals.
- Create a positive and inclusive school climate where all students feel safe.
- Improve attendance and punctuality of all students across the school.

Cognitive-Based Regulation Programs

Cognitive regulation is an aspect of executive functioning that allows children to control aspects of their thoughts to attend, plan, execute, socialize, and perform daily activities (Schunk & DiBenedetto, 2020). It differs from sensory regulation in that it is a higher-level cognitive function that occurs in the brain's cortical areas and requires the frontal lobe to inhibit and make judgment calls. Cognitive regulation is important for all children. However, when children have sensory processing differences, cognitive regulation is often insufficient to maintain attention, focus, and control impulses. Cognition can override sensory processing to a point, meaning that students can use cognition to regulate their sensory needs. Yet, for children with sensory processing differences, often their sensory needs become too much to override or reason through cognitively. When the body has an unfilled sensory need, or the body needs particular sensory input to maintain a state of homeostasis, cognition can be used to ignore these sensory needs until the body reaches such a state of imbalance that the ability to reason is not enough to outweigh the need to achieve homeostasis. At that point, the child must receive the sensory input needed for homeostasis. Often, they will do anything to meet this need, whether that attempt is adaptive or maladaptive.

However, the use of cognitive regulation is key in the overall development of self-awareness, executive functioning, adaptive behaviors, and social interaction. Sensory regulation is one of the three aspects that impact self-regulation overall. Those three areas include cognitive regulation, an aspect of executive functioning, emotional regulation, and finally, sensory regulation. Children need to develop all three areas to have mature regulation (Kuypers, 2011). Connecting sensory needs and sensory regulation to emotional and cognitive regulation can help children develop the necessary skills needed for mature regulation and social interactions.

There are many commercially available cognitive regulation programs that focus on regulating sensory systems. These programs may be designed for the individual but can easily be implemented at a population or group level, and vice versa. The following section will discuss three cognitive-based sensory regulation programs. For full details on each program, the implementer should read the program manuals and implementation guides. This section only presents an overview of the program and focuses on implementing the programs at the Tier 1 and Tier 2 levels.

In cognitive-based sensory regulation programs, there is no good or bad level. This contrasts behavioral regulation programs that frequently distinguish behavioral levels as being positive or negative. In sensory regulation programs, there is the assumption that each task requires a different level of alertness or arousal, and people are expected to move between all levels of alertness at different times throughout the day. The need for sensory regulation occurs when there is a mismatch between the level of alertness and the task demands. It is then that regulation strategies must be initiated to modify the alertness level to match the task.

The Alert Program

The Alert Program® was developed by Mary Sue Williams and Shelly Shellenberger (2025). It is also known as *How Does Your Engine Run?* and is one of the earliest published curriculums for cognitive-based sensory regulation. The program presents three levels of alertness, much as a car engine runs at low, just right, and high speeds. The idea is that each person has an internal engine that runs at different speeds throughout the day, just as a car runs at different speeds during a journey. Continuing with the car metaphor, a car has a speedometer to indicate variations between speeds based on how much gas is given to the car or when brakes are applied. Self-regulation strategies provide more "gas" or less "gas" to change the alertness level, sometimes slightly and sometimes more extreme, just as when the brakes are applied in a car. Many therapists have modified this program to utilize other images that describe the different levels of alertness. The instructional manual that accompanies the program provides many examples and a full curriculum. The program manual provides a group curriculum that can easily be implemented at the Tier 1 and Tier 2 levels.

Zones of Regulation

Zones of Regulation is a program by Leah M. Kuypers (2011). It was initially part of the Social Thinking curriculum (Winner, 2007). This program combines sensory and emotional regulation, tying emotions and sensory processing together in four levels of alertness. The "blue" level is the lower alertness level and is tied to emotions such as sadness, tiredness, and loneliness. A child in this level may be under stimulated from a sensory processing standpoint. The "green" level is equivalent to the "just right" level in the Alert Program. It is tied to emotions such as happiness, calm, and alertness. At this level, the child's sensory needs are fulfilled, and their body is ready to attend to and complete schoolwork or social activities. The "yellow" level is a higher level of alertness but not to the point of overstimulation or feeling out of control. It includes emotions such as nervousness, excitement, silliness, and worry. Some tasks and activities require a "yellow" level for optimum participation. For example, a child going to an amusement park would be expected to be in the "yellow" zone due to excitement. The "red" zone represents extreme feelings that are often overwhelming. These include feelings of elation, rage, panic, and euphoria. It is often a feeling of being out of control. The "red" zone is not a time when the brain's cognitive areas can process very much cognitive information other than the experience of the emotion at the time. The child is often in a state of survival, not in a state of thinking and reasoning. It is important to help a child decrease their level of alertness before cognitively processing the situation and emotion. Figure 5.5 provides a sample of wall posters that can be used to help students match emotions and levels of alertness to various zones.

The concept of expected and unexpected behaviors is part of the *Social Thinking* curriculum (Winner, 2007). It takes away the idea that emotions or reactions are good or bad. Instead, the reaction, feeling, or behavior is expected or unexpected in certain situations. This depends upon various environmental factors, including the physical and social environment and task demands. The concept of expected or unexpected reactions or behaviors removes the idea that emotions are negative or that we should not experience or feel certain emotions. It allows a child to experience and process emotions without adding the additional emotion of negativity. The child can begin to understand emotions and reactions and how feelings, emotions, and responses to emotions impact the environment. Identifying and naming emotions helps a child understand emotional regulation and develop inhibitory control. Inhibitory control allows a child to interact with the environment successfully when things happen as expected and when they do not happen as expected (Chowdhury, 2019).

The *Zones of Regulation* curriculum has become common at the Tier 1 level in many schools. It is a great tool for encouraging social development and helping students learn how to regulate sensory processing and emotions within the school setting. However, it can often be misused as a behavioral program, which is different from the intention of the program. Many school personnel revert to their understanding of behavioral modification based on positive behavioral support and reinforcement. This perception is embedded, albeit incorrectly, in the presentation of the *Zones of Regulation*. As a result, the program is utilized

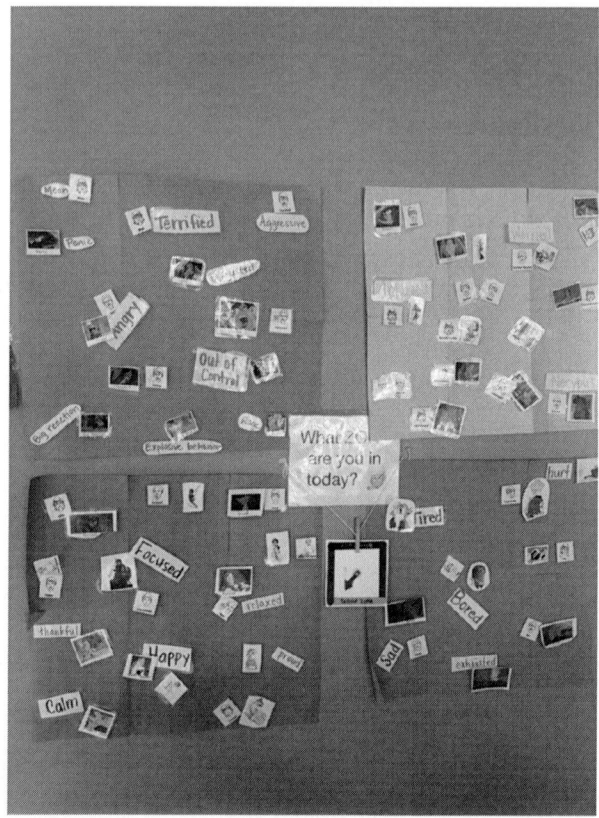

Figure 5.5 Sample wall posters based on Zones of Regulation (Kuypers, 2011). Image by author.

as a behavior program, which may consider one zone better or more accept-able than another. This directly contradicts the original curriculum of Zones of Regulation, which emphasizes that children should experience each zone at dif-ferent points. When implementing this program at a Tier 1 level, staff training is key so that school personnel understand and reinforce the program as a sensory and emotional regulation program rather than a behavioral program.

The curriculum is designed for implementation in groups, including small groups and larger groups. It is divided into lessons with time for instruction and learning activities. As written, it can be used at Tier 1 and Tier 2 levels.

Sensory Ladders

Sensory Ladders was developed by Kath Smith (2001) based on the PEO model and was designed to support Ayres Sensory Integration®. It was initially developed for adults but has since been modified for use with all ages. The goal of this program is to help participants have a better understanding of their personal sensory and emotional systems. This program provides a visual aid representing different emotional, sensory, and physical levels. These levels range from low to high and illustrate how sensory input can affect a child's state of alertness, arousal, and emotion. The visual is set up as a ladder with rungs that represent a different state or feeling. This can help students identify and articulate how they feel at different times of the day and with different activities. While the ladder is the original visual concept, children may generate any picture that they desire to represent their personalized level of feelings and arousal. Each level is labeled with a sensory and emotional descriptor. Typically, these labels are similar to low arousal, calm, alert, agitated, and overwhelmed, but can be any variation of those terms. The student can represent each rung however they choose to help them identify their current emotional or sensory state. Students should then generate a list of coping strategies to use at each level of the ladder. The following are examples of sensory and emotional descriptors and accompanying coping strategies.

- **Low arousal (tired, bored)**: Activities that increase alertness, such as physical exercise or listening to upbeat music.
- **Optimal arousal (calm, focused)**: Consistent routines, sensory breaks to maintain level.
- **High arousal (anxious or agitated)**: Activities to calm, such as deep pressure or quiet time.

Students should consistently refer to the ladder to identify their level of alertness and practice implementing various activities and strategies as their alertness levels change. They can add and change activities as warranted. While the ladder is commonly used, students may choose to use any figure or image to represent their own feelings. Figure 5.6 provides a sample of a student's sensory ladder in the shape of a caterpillar.

Sensory Ladders is a very individualized program, but it can still be utilized at Tier 1 and Tier 2 levels. As a class or group, students can work together to develop a ladder, working collaboratively to describe and generate a list of activities to use at each level that can be implemented into their classroom routines easily. These can be posted for the class or group to see and use as needed. It also allows students to monitor one another in an attempt to promote independence in emotional and sensory regulation. In addition, students can develop an individualized ladder to accompany the classroom or small group ladder with more individualized strategies they can implement as needed.

Now, let us see how we can practically implement these interventions at both Tier 1 and 2 levels.

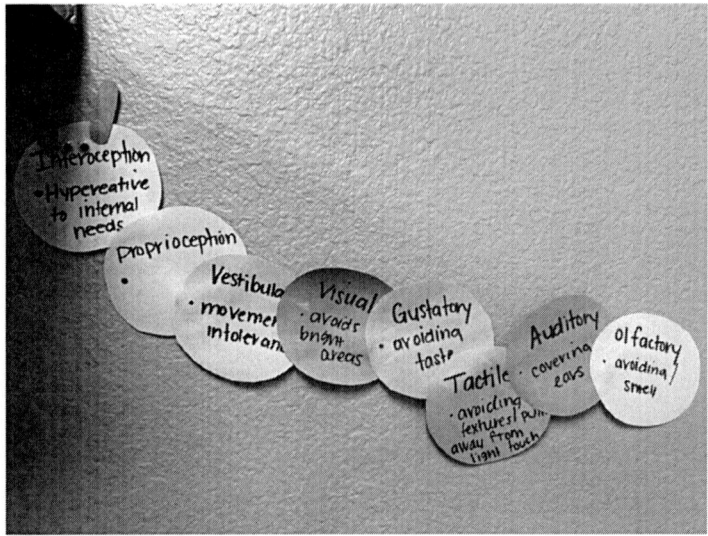

Figure 5.6 A student's sensory ladder in the shape of a caterpillar.

Bringing it Together

Tier 1

When working with schools and classrooms at a Tier 1 level, the occupational therapist should first address the environment. The population assessment will guide the occupational therapist toward what needs to be implemented and when, but the first step is changes to the environment, including routines. The occupational therapist should consider the visual environment, auditory environment, and access to other sensory activities. Providing other sensory activities such as a fidget box, alternative seating, and a sensory station with tactile and proprioceptive activities is an excellent way to modify the environment to increase the match between the class and the environment to promote participation. The occupational therapist should also help the teacher design routines that are more conducive to learning and provide opportunities for calming input and alerting input based on the tasks of the day. For example, adding a 15-minute yoga session directly after lunch and recess to help the students organize and calm for the afternoon. If students are in an organized state, this will help them remain organized to complete their afternoon seat work. Next, the occupational therapist can implement a cognitive-based self-regulation program. This will help staff and students learn their sensory needs and guide staff in promoting self-regulation. Staff should be trained in the program and demonstrate competence

Table 5.5 Sample Sensory Intervention Plan for Tier 1

Intervention area	Tier 1 Interventions
Sensory environment	**Visual**: Light covers and shades to dim the lighting **Auditory**: Quiet corner **Tactile**: Fidget box available to all students **Vestibular**: Students can choose alternative seating options such as standing, ball chairs, t-stool, etc. **Deep pressure**: provide a basket of weighted items, such as lap pads, blankets, etc. that can be accessed and used as needed
Classroom routines	Students participate in movement sequences in the morning consisting of windmills, jumping jacks, and arm squeezes After lunch and recess students participate in classroom-wide yoga for 15 minutes to provide weight-bearing and heavy work to organize for the afternoon
Cognitive-sensory regulation	Perform an in-service session before school starts, where the teachers and classroom assistants are trained in Sensory Ladders; the occupation therapist facilitates a classroom group for students to design their sensory ladder, which the teacher posts and allows students to add activities to throughout the year
Sensory input	Design a small section of the classroom with pillows, a sensory bin, a therapy ball, and exercises posted on the wall; students can access this area throughout the day to get the sensory input they need Design a sensory walk in the hallway with animal walks, hops, break stations with exercises, etc., that teachers can utilize when students are transitioning between environments

in implementation before initiation of the program. Finally, implementing sensory stations within the classroom or sensory walks within the school's hallways is an excellent way to increase sensory input throughout the day for all students. Table 5.5 provides an example of a Tier 1 sensory intervention plan.

Figure 5.7 shows a table with four different types of seating options for students. This is an example of a Tier 1 sensory environmental modification to provide multiple alternative seating options for students who may need additional movement when seated.

Tier 2

Tier 2 interventions are more targeted to a group of students who have identified sensory needs. When implementing Tier 2 interventions, students can be grouped based on their sensory processing patterns. For example, children with more hyperreactive responses to sensory input can be grouped with students

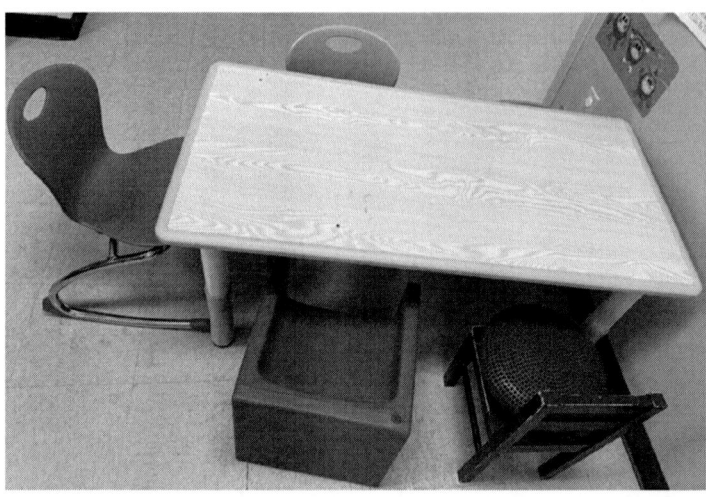

Figure 5.7 Samples of alternative seating at one table, showing an example of a Tier 1
intervention. Image by author.

with similar sensory processing patterns. Groups of students can be from the
same or different classrooms, based on the structure of the school. Tier 1 interventions should continue even when Tier 2 interventions have been initiated, so
interventions performed at Tier 2 can be more individualized implementations
of Tier 1 sensory interventions.

Under Tier 2, smaller environments can be created within the classroom that
are conducive to the needs of groups of students. For example, an area with
decreased lighting, no strong scents, and noise-dampening items on the wall
can create a quieter space for students to work with less sensory stimulation.
On the other hand, for students who need more sensory stimulation, a visually
vibrant area with background music and diffusers to provide calming scents can
be designed for students who may be more hyporeactive to sensory input. Under
Tier 2 students would have their own alternative seating available at their work
area, rather than just having seating options available for the class.

Additional modifications to the seating area can be made, such as Velcro on
the bottom of the desk, fidgets kept in the desk, or resistance bands around the
legs of the desk or chair for increased proprioceptive input. Providing specific
times during the day for sensory breaks or movement groups can provide needed
sensory input to students under Tier 2 at the times they most need the input to
be at the optimal alertness. Sensory breaks can be designed to provide either
alerting or organizing input or a combination of both types of input based on
the group of students' needs. Movement groups may consist of yoga groups,

Table 5.6 Tier 2 Intervention Plan

Type of Intervention	Intervention
Sensory environment	Create low-stimulation areas and higher-stimulation areas for students who need less or more sensory input; based on their sensory needs, design a schedule for students to use these areas
Classroom routines	Embed sensory groups within classroom routines when the group of students needs additional sensory input, either calming or alerting based on the group's sensory needs; this may mean there are times the group exits the classroom to engage in sensory activities, or the students may be provided a schedule of the best times to utilize sensory-based interventions (i.e. weighted items, headphones, etc.) and lower/higher stimulation areas
Cognitive-sensory regulation	Provide additional instruction time for the cognitive-based curriculum implemented in Tier 1 or implement a cognitive-sensory regulation program as a small group program
Sensory input	Small groups are designed with the students' needs in mind; design movement groups or obstacle courses to meet sensory needs; provide sensory tools based on the students' needs, such as alternative seating, weighted items, and fidgets that are kept at the students' workstations to be used when they need them

dance groups, running groups, and obstacle courses designed to meet the sensory needs of the group of students. If the school or classroom has not implemented a cognitive-based sensory regulation program, any of the programs listed above can be implemented within small groups. If cognitive-sensory regulation programs are implemented at Tier 1, students receiving Tier 2 support should spend additional time on the programs to create more customized approaches to cognitive sensory regulation. You can see an example intervention plan for a Tier 2 group in Table 5.6.

Summary

Providing sensory interventions at Tier 1 and Tier 2 levels can help many students regulate and attend during the school day. While all students have varying sensory processing needs, the occupational therapist can utilize general principles of sensory processing to design interventions that address barriers to participation that were identified in the evaluation. The occupational therapist can work with the students and teachers to build upon sensory processing strengths implementing an evidence-based intervention such as PEO, ASI, or EHP to guide the intervention process. The occupational therapist can consider the sensory environment and various ways to modify the sensory environment to meet the needs of students within that environment. In addition, sensory activities designed to impact arousal levels can be designed within the school's routines to help ensure student's sensory needs are met, their arousal levels match the task demands, and they have a supportive sensory environment. Finally, occupational therapists can implement cognitive-based sensory regulation strategies that help students understand their own sensory processing and how sensory processing impacts levels of arousal, and prompts independence implementing sensory strategies to support participation in academic activities.

By delivering high-quality interventions based on evidence, theory, and assessment results, students can meet their sensory needs while participating in classroom learning activities and routines. Assessing sensory needs and providing customized intervention plans allows for skilled occupational therapy services to be provided at Tier 1 and Tier 2 levels that intervene before students require more direct and intensive sensory support services.

Chapter 6 will now cover how to assess sensory interventions and gather quality data to determine if interventions are effective in meeting goals and supporting progress for students.

References

American Occupational Therapy Association (AOTA) (2020). Occupational therapy practice framework: Domain and process–Fourth edition. *American Journal of Occupational Therapy, 74*(S2), 1–85. https://doi.org/10.5014/ajot.2020.74S2001.

Ayres, A. J. (1979). *Sensory Integration and the Child.* Western Psychological Services.

Bundy, A. C. & Lane, S. J. (2020). Sensory integration: A. Jean Ayres' theory revisited. In A. C. Bundy & S. J. Lane (eds), *Sensory Integration Theory and Practice*, 3rd ed., pp. 2–20. F. A. Davis.

Case-Smith, J., Weaver, L. L., & Fristad, M. A. (2015). A systematic review of sensory processing interventions for children with autism spectrum disorders. *Autism, 19*(2), 133–148. https://doi.org/10.1177/1362361313517762.

CDC Physical Activity Basics (2024). *What you can do to meet the physical activity recommendations.* https://www.cdc.gov/physical-activity-basics/guidelines/index.html

Chowdhury, M. R. (2019). *Emotional Regulation: 6 Key Skills to Regulate Emotions.* https://positivepsychology.com/emotion-regulation/.

Dunn, W., Brown, C., & McGuigan, A. (1994). The ecology of human performance: A framework for considering the effect of context. *American Journal of Occupational Therapy, 48*(7), 595–607. https://doi.org/10.5014/ajot.48.7.595.

Fernández-Andrés, M. I., Pastor-Cerezuela, G., Sanz-Cervera, P., & Tárraga-Mínguez, R. (2015). A comparative study of sensory processing in children with and without autism spectrum disorder in the home and classroom environments. *Research in Developmental Disabilities, 38*, 202–212. doi: 10.1016/j.ridd.2014.12.034.

Ikuta, N., Iwanaga, R., Tokunaga, A., Nakane, H., Tanaka, K., & Tanaka, G. (2016). Effectiveness of earmuffs and noise-cancelling headphones for coping with hyperreactivity to auditory stimuli in children with autism spectrum disorder: A preliminary study. *Hong Kong Journal of Occupational Therapy*, *28*(1), 24–32. https://doi.org/10.1016/j.hkjot.2016.09.001.

Koepp, A. E., Gershoff, E. T., Castelli, D. M., & Bryan, A. E. (2022). Preschoolers' executive functions following indoor and outdoor free play. *Trends in Neuroscience and Education*, *28*, 100182. https://doi.org/10.1016/j.tine.2022.100182.

Kuypers, L. (2011). *The Zones of Regulation.* Social Thinking Publishing.

Law, M., Cooper, B., Strong, S., Stewart, D., Rigby, P., & Letts, L. (1996). The person-environment-occupation model: A transactive approach to occupational performance. *Canadian Journal of Occupational Therapy*, *63*(1), 9–23. https://doi.org/10.1177/000841749606300103.

Parham, L. D., Roley, S. S., May-Benson, T. A., Koomar, J., Brett-Green, B., Burke, J. P., Cohn, E. S., Mailloux, Z., Miller, L. J., & Schaaf, R. C. (2011). Development of a fidelity measure for research on the effectiveness of the Ayres Sensory Integration® intervention. *American Journal of Occupational Therapy*, *65*(2), 133–142. https://doi.org/10.5014/ajot.2011.000745.

Schaaf, R. C. & Mailloux, Z. (2015). *Clinician's Guide for Implementing Ayres Sensory Integration®: Promoting Participation for Children with Autism.* AOTA Press.

Schunk, D. & DiBenedetto, M. (2020, May 29). Cognitive Regulation. *Oxford Research Encyclopedia of Education.* https://oxfordre.com/education/view/10.1093/acrefore/9780190264093.001.0001/acrefore-9780190264093-e-886.

Smith, K (2001). *Sensory Ladders for Self-Regulation.* https://sensoryladders.org/.

Whiting, C. C., Schoen, S. A., & Niemeyer, L. (2023). A sensory integration intervention in the school setting to support performance and participation: A multiple-baseline study. *American Journal of Occupational Therapy*, *77*(2), 7702205060. https://doi.org/10.5014/ajot.2023.050135.

Williams, M. S. and Shellenberger S. (2025). *"How Does Your Engine Run?" A Leader's Guide to the Alert Program for Self-Regulation.* (2nd Edition) Therapy Works, Inc.

Winner, M. G. (2007) *Thinking About You, Thinking About Me.* Think Social Publishing, Inc.

Evaluating Outcomes of Interventions

Introduction

So far, along with understanding how sensory processing can impact education, we have explored and examined how to assess and design interventions for children with sensory processing needs in the school setting. However, without evaluating whether these interventions are actually helping the children access learning at Tier 1 or Tier 2 levels, this work is, at best, redundant or, at worst, potentially harmful to the students. Further, evaluating progress is a requirement of a multi-tiered system of supports (MTSS). Progress monitoring methods must be valid and reliable, utilizing repeated measures over time to evaluate progress (American Institutes for Research [AIR], 2023).

Therefore, this chapter will discuss the importance of monitoring the outcomes of provided interventions to ensure they promote learning and access to the curriculum, and support participation in the academic setting. In addition, this chapter will offer common methods of gathering high-quality data and explain how to use this data to modify interventions if needed. Finally, this chapter briefly discusses discharge planning from a higher tier to a lower tier, providing guidance on how to ensure necessary supports are provided at a lower tier if warranted.

Importance of Outcomes

Clearly defined outcomes are an essential part of the occupational therapy process, and they should be considered as soon as the occupational therapy process is initiated (American Occupational Therapy Association [AOTA], 2020). Outcomes help determine the need for occupational therapy and allow the therapist to measure progress and determine if interventions are effective, which is required under the MTSS model. Although many districts have their own established procedures for monitoring and collecting data, it is important to consider different methods of deciding outcome measures. In addition to this, outcomes are essential for helping occupational therapists to gather data according to best

DOI: 10.4324/9781032654768-7

practice, interpret outcomes to make informed decisions on modification and continuation of interventions, and plan for discharge.

The first step in defining outcomes is the evaluation, which provides baseline data. The clear baseline allows for a point of reference to compare future outcomes and evaluate the effectiveness of interventions. By repeating the same assessment at a later date, outcomes can be compared to the initial data to show change and growth.

Occupational therapy practitioners need to consider several factors when choosing outcome measures. First, the outcome measure needs to be valid, reliable, and sensitive to change to show progress over time. The outcome measure needs to be targeted at identified goals and predictive of future outcomes (American Occupational Therapy Organization [AOTA], 2020). Goal attainment or achievement is one method of measuring progress while ensuring that outcomes are centered around what is meaningful to the client. This is often done in the school setting through progress monitoring. At the group level, outcomes may look at the effectiveness of interventions and how individuals within a group interact. For example, when implementing a sensory group, the occupational therapist may consider the social dynamics of the group while addressing the overall group goal of improving behavior and social participation. At the population level, outcomes may address concepts of self-advocacy, integration of students within the classroom system, and accessing needed sensory input during the school day (AOTA, 2020).

Outcomes can be standardized assessments or unstructured evaluation methods via formal and informal means. It is good practice for the occupational therapist to continuously utilize a combination of formal and informal outcomes during the occupational therapy process. Let us take a look at these different types of formal and informal assessments and their considerations.

Norm-Referenced Assessments

The occupational therapist must consider many factors when choosing outcome measures, including a general understanding of the types of outcomes, their psychometric properties, and the importance of clinical utility. Standardized measures may be norm-referenced or criterion-referenced. Normed reference assessments compare and rank the client to others who have taken the same assessment, which is known as the normative sample. The Bell Curve is commonly referred to in normed reference assessments, as it represents the normal distribution of the sample. The curve provides standard deviations, which refer to the distribution of scores around the mean and define the variation in data. Scores are expected to fall within certain ranges of the median score in a normal distribution (Griswold, 2014).

Students are often compared to a normative population using standardized educational assessment data. This information is frequently used to determine service eligibility, especially when evaluating students at the Tier 3 level. Many districts may have established criteria to qualify for services at the Tier 3 level, which is based on normative data on standardized assessments. For example, a district may require a student to fall at least two standard deviations below the mean to qualify for occupational therapy services. Since occupational therapy is a related service rather than an eligibility category, districts may leave the decision-making of eligibility for occupational therapy services in the hands of the evaluating occupational therapist rather than having set cut-off eligibility criteria. Many normed referenced assessments are designed to be used as pre/post-intervention outcomes to measure change. However, not all assessments are designed to show change over time, so the evaluating therapist should consult the assessment manual for more information.

Criterion-Referenced Assessments

Criterion-referenced assessments compare clients to a set standard or criteria. These assessments may also use predetermined cut scores to categorize assessment takers. This is common in educational settings where students may be placed into categories such as basic, emergent, proficient, or advanced. With a criterion-referenced assessment, the number of students scoring at a certain level is irrelevant. The only relevance of a score is to a set of pre-established criteria (Griswold, 2014). Many self-report or observer-reported assessments are criterion-referenced.

Psychometric Properties

Psychometric properties of assessments need to be considered when determining which assessments best suit the client and the outcomes being measured. The concepts essential to psychometric properties consist of reliability, which refers to the stability of the assessment over time, and validity, which refers to the concept being measured and whether the assessment truly measures the concept it intends to measure. In addition, clinicians should consider the floor and ceiling effect and clinical utility of the instrument.

Most assessments provide information on psychometric properties in the test manual, which clinicians must review before deciding whether to implement an assessment for a chosen outcome. In the school setting, one of the criteria under the Individuals with Disabilities Education Act (IDEA) for assessments utilized in an evaluation process for special education services is that assessments must be reliable and valid tests. Therefore, occupational therapists working in the school setting must have a solid understanding of reliability and validity regarding the student, setting, and purpose they are evaluating. We will now take a closer look at both of these considerations.

Reliability

When choosing an evaluation method, the common types of reliability which occupational therapists should consider are interrater, internal consistency, and test/retest reliability.

Interrater reliability measures the agreement of different test administrators or raters for the same assessment. When a test has a high interrater reliability, it means that results remain consistent regardless of who administers the assessment (Portney, 2020). In the school setting, there may be many different raters for one student, so high interrater reliability is important. In addition, when addressing sensory processing differences, outcomes are often composed of various behaviors that can be subjective to evaluate. Ensuring outcome measures have high interrater reliability allows any trained professional to gather outcome data with the assurance that it is consistent with the original evaluator.

Internal consistency examines the extent to which items in an assessment measure a single construct or idea. It demonstrates whether the tool measures the intended concept and not a variety of concepts or unintended concepts (Portney 2020). For example, when evaluating sensory reactivity, an assessment with high internal consistency would show it was assessing sensory reactivity and not adaptive/maladaptive behaviors.

Test-retest reliability examines the consistency of the assessment to maintain the same results over a period of time. Test-retest reliability is often determined with a two-week gap between the first and second administration, and the goal is that the results remain consistent over time. Of course, many factors can impact results, and often factors are outside the control of the administrator or test taker. An outcome with high test-retest reliability indicates that these extraneous factors do not significantly affect the assessment results (Portney, 2020). When considering repeated measures of the same assessment, it is important to examine test-retest reliability and whether the instrument was designed to be used as an outcome measure. Some assessments demonstrate good responsiveness, meaning the tool is designed to measure and capture change over time. A tool with high responsiveness may be a good choice for an outcome measure to assess change over time.

Validity

Validity, in a nutshell, indicates that an assessment measures what it intends to assess. There are many different methods to measure validity, and these methods are typically described in detail in the assessment manual. Additionally, they often involve comparisons to other previously standardized assessments (Portney, 2020).

For occupational therapists, there are four main types of validity to consider: content, construct, concurrent, and predictive.

- **Content validity** means the assessment utilizes the correct aspects to measure what it intends to measure.
- **Construct validity** means the assessment measures what it set out to measure.
- **Concurrent validity** refers to the ability of the assessment to measure something else that is also being measured.
- **Predictive validity** refers to measuring something that may occur in the future.

Often, the evaluation report contains a statement of validity. Hence, evaluators must ensure they review this portion of the manual and include it in the assessment write-up.

Floor and Ceiling Effects

Floor and ceiling effects are the results of extreme lows and highs of scores. If an instrument has a floor effect, it may not effectively show differences in students that score very low on the scale. With ceiling effects, a student with a very high score may not demonstrate any change. In both cases of extreme low and high scores, small changes may not be detected in that assessment (Portney, 2020). Consideration of floor and ceiling effects are important if the occupational therapist needs to show a change in performance for students that may score very low or very high on an assessment.

Clinical Utility

Clinical utility refers to how useful an assessment is in practice. Assessments with high clinical utility provide reliable and valid information that supports and guides practice, and provide information to inform clinical reasoning. As a result, interventions are more likely to produce positive outcomes (Badrick & Bowling, 2023). While clinical utility may be subjective, it is important to consider how the assessment informs the intervention plan. Using theory-based assessments can help ensure clinical utility in occupational therapy.

Types of Outcomes

Occupational therapists can use many types of outcomes to gather data about the effectiveness of interventions and determine the next course of action. When deciding whether to modify or continue an intervention, goal attainment, goal achievement, and progress toward goals are common outcome measures in occupational therapy. Within the school setting, outcomes can be either reported or observed through formal and informal questionnaires and standardized assessments, which we will now review.

Self/Caregiver/Teacher Report

When working with children, many outcomes are often self-reported or reported by proxy, with a teacher or aide reporting on behalf of the child. Some examples of standardized reports regarding sensory processing include the Sensory Processing Measure-2 (SPM-2) (Parham et al., 2021) and the Sensory Profile-2 (SP-2) (Dunn, 2014), both of which have a school and home version to allow parents and school personnel to report about the child.

While gaining the teacher and caregiver perspective is key, it is also important to gather information about the child from the child. Even if the child is young, understanding how the child views and processes sensory information is important in assessing outcomes and changes resulting from an intervention. The Sensory and Satisfaction Questionnaire (Stansberry & Piller, 2023) is a child report measure designed to gain information on a child's sensory processing and satisfaction with interventions for children as young as three years of age. When using self- or proxy-reported outcomes, it is important to ensure they are designed to be used as an outcome measure. Many of the sensory questionnaires are not designed to measure progress and may show a decrease in scores as the person who is reporting starts to understand more about sensory processing. Further, sensory processing often fluctuates, and many sensory reactivity assessments (i.e. SPM-2 and SP2) are designed to reflect the changes in sensory processing rather than the effectiveness of interventions. In other words, they were not designed to be outcome measures.

It may be beneficial for the occupational therapist to develop a self- or teacher report that targets the exact areas of improvement as stated in the goals. This could be achieved by using one of the following.

- **Likert scales**: Often five- or seven-point scales that are an excellent way to provide quick feedback and demonstrate whether interventions are effective.
- **Frequency counts**: These are an easy way to measure progress for identified behaviors.
- **Standard forms for teachers and other school personnel**: These can help the occupational therapist gain quality data on targeted outcomes.

Performance-Based

Performance-based outcomes ask a student to perform a particular set of tasks or demonstrate specific behaviors. They can be objective and quantifiable through measures such as time, assistance level needed, or simply checking if a skill is present or absent. Examples of performance-based sensory assessments include the Structured Observations of Sensory Integration-Motor (SOSI-M) (Blanche et al., 2021), the Goal-Oriented Assessment of Life Skills (Miller et al., 2013), or the Evaluation in Ayres Sensory Integration® (EASI) (Mailloux et al., 2018). These involve the child performing various tasks that are observed and rated by the testing administrator.

Observer Reported

In occupational therapy, the therapist can observe and provide information on anticipated and preset outcomes. The importance of using clinician-observed observations is that the occupational therapy practitioner is able to implement their professional understanding and reasoning regarding sensory processing in the observation. This allows for additional information and understanding of measured outcomes that others may not fully understand or know when making observations. An example of an assessment that utilizes an observer report is the Short Child Occupational Profile (SCOPE) (Bowyer et al., 2008). The SCOPE allows for the evaluating occupational therapist to use a variety of methods to rate a child's occupational performance, volition, and habituation, one of which is observation. This assessment provides a method to evaluate occupational performance and has the flexibility to combine observation, interview, and performance into one rating. However, if the occupational therapist is only able to use one of the methods, such as observation, this also produces a valid assessment. Further, this assessment provides an assessment of the environment, which can be used to provide information on if the environment is a facilitator or barrier to participation, thus allowing the occupational therapist to know if an environmental modification would be warranted.

Program Outcomes

Program outcomes refer to the desired goals of the school or district through the implementation of the MTSS framework. Program outcomes tend to be holistic and include things such as improved academic performance, improved positive behavior, increased student engagement, improved school climate, and efficient use of resources (AIR, 2024). The implementation of sensory interventions can support many desired program outcomes of a school and district. The successful implementation of sensory supports through Tier 1 and Tier 2 has the potential to improve academic achievement for students. When students are regulated from a sensory processing standpoint, they are better able to use their cognitive and executive functioning skills to participate in academic activities, organize their assignments to complete on time, and improve academic performance. Further, when students are regulated, they can manage their behaviors better and participate more effectively in social tasks. Therefore, the successful implementation of sensory interventions at all MTSS levels can support overall positive program outcomes.

Universal screenings are a key component of MTSS to identify students that may need additional support or are at risk of falling behind in academics, behavior, or social and emotional engagement. Universal screenings are performed on a regular basis and should have clear goals as to who is to be identified through the screening process. An example of target populations includes identifying students who need additional resources or those who are at risk for poor academic outcomes (AIR, 2024). Successful universal screening programs also include structured methods to gather and track data in order to accurately identify students with needs and what those needs may be in relation to the set goals (Missal et al., 2021). The occupational therapist can and should be part of the universal screening process for two main reasons. First, universal screenings related to sensory needs provide the needed information to tailor a Tier 1 sensory-based school-wide intervention. Second, universal screening helps the occupational therapist be aware of students who may need special attention or increased intervention support in the future. In this way, key sensory or behavioral indicators can be part of the screening process to assess whether students need more support with their sensory processing.

Under universal screening, the occupational therapist would screen all students based on specific indicators determined by the district or school, and they should be part of the planning process to implement and administer universal screenings. When selecting a tool for universal screening of sensory needs, the occupational therapist should consider brief assessments that can be performed and analyzed quickly and efficiently for all students. Universal screeners may provide criterion and norm reference results, or they may just provide quantitative data that the school team can analyze to determine progress and effectiveness. The assessments for universal screening are typically performed at specified intervals throughout the school year. Hence, it is important to pay attention to the tool's psychometric properties and how often it can be re-administered.

When occupational therapists help design or implement a universal screening procedure, they must work with the MTSS team to ensure effective and efficient methods of gathering quality data. During the universal screening process, frequency counts are an easy way to generate data, provide baselines, and track progress quickly. Tracking the frequency of particular behaviors associated with sensory processing differences can allow occupational therapists to monitor progress and help identify students who need additional support. The data set can be analyzed as a whole, indicating the number of times any student demonstrated the behavior or the data can be analyzed by student, with averages provided. These can show change over time and provide data for implementing sensory supports. The decisions on how best to analyze the data are up to the MTSS team and should align with the goals and baseline data.

Here are some potential behaviors to track using frequency counts.

- On-task behavior/time on task.
- Number of tasks completed in a given amount of time.
- Getting up from seat.
- Sensory avoiding behaviors such as hands over ears, covering eyes, etc.
- Avoidance of tasks.
- Eloping behaviors/leaving the environment.
- Aggression toward other students.
- Times student raised hand and waited to be called on.
- Positive initiated interactions with peers during group discussions.

In addition, the occupational therapist may want to gather data from the teacher and students through a survey or observations during the universal screening process. A Likert scale can easily be used to gather data and monitor progress. Here is an example of a Likert scale.

- 1: Rarely or never (less than one time per day).
- 2: Occasionally (one or two times per day).
- 3: Frequently (several times per day).
- 4: Almost always (many times a day such that it interrupts the flow of the class).

Here are a few sample survey questions that can be used with the Likert scale.

- How often do you have to decrease the lighting or sound in your classroom to help students pay attention or stay on task?
- How often do you find the students in your classroom need additional movement other than physical education and recess?
- How often do you have to ask students to remain on task?
- How often do you find students engaging in rough play or interactions with other students?
- How often do students raise their hands and wait to be called on?
- How often do you provide prompts when it is time to quiet down and attend the lecture or work?

Keeping Interventions Student-Centered

Occupational therapy practitioners are concerned with clients' needs, values, and preferences. They seek to incorporate a client-centered care model that views the client as a partner in the therapy process. In this way, occupational therapy practitioners use professional reasoning to embed client-centered interventions and outcomes throughout occupational therapy (AOTA, 2020). Under this model, the client has choice and autonomy (Schell & Gillen, 2019) and should be intricately involved in each phase of the occupational therapy process. When working with children, occupational therapy practitioners should be mindful to not only rely on what caregivers and teachers indicate is important. The skilled occupational therapy practitioner will ensure that the child's perspective and needs are at the center of the intervention process and that the student plays a role within it.

A critical aspect of student-centered interventions is ensuring students are part of the evaluation and feedback process. The use of interviews, questionnaires, and small group discussions can allow students to provide feedback directly to the occupational therapist rather than only from proxy sources, such as teachers and assistants. The occupational therapist can make changes based on student feedback, ensuring these changes fit within the guidelines of the setting where the intervention occurs. In addition, occupational therapy practitioners should promote neuro-affirming approaches to interventions, working with a student's strengths rather than viewing the student from a deficit model.

Special education services in the school setting have historically been focused on a deficit intervention model. However, with the implementation of MTSS came the opportunity to function from a neuro-affirming approach. Under the MTSS model, barriers to universal learning can be addressed and removed to allow all learners to succeed. Neuro-affirming approaches to learning focus on strengths rather than deficits. In addition, neuro-affirming interventions are collaborative with students, ensuring they have a voice in the process. They focus on fostering a partnership between teachers, occupational therapy practitioners, and students to ensure there is a cohesive support system that addresses the holistic needs of many learners, both neurodiverse and neurotypical. Under this model, school personnel work hard to eliminate environmental and attitudinal barriers that may prevent diverse learners from meeting their sensory needs and maximizing their learning.

The school staff helps students build confidence and self-esteem by ensuring the interventions are student-centered. Student-centered approaches offer choices for all learners, and school personnel help facilitate choices that meet the needs of the student, the goals of the student, and the learning goals of the classroom. Supports are viewed as positive in helping students become the students they want to be and reach their academic potential. Students must be valued for their identity and not pressured to fit into a specified mold. By providing a variety of sensory spaces in the classroom and school and making sensory tools available to all students under an MTSS Tier 1 model, the school makes steps towards a student-centered, neuro-affirming environment. Students should be allowed to meet their sensory needs when required and have access to a sensory environment conducive to their learning. Students can engage in self-advocacy as they learn more about themselves and their personal sensory needs. The occupational therapist can support the development of self-advocacy skills by constantly gaining feedback from students rather than just relying on the teacher's report of their sensory processing and regulation. Offering tracking sheets that students can complete independently is one way to gain student feedback and regularly engage in progress monitoring. Remember, even young students can provide input via pictures or words. The use of images, such as smiley faces, may be a nice alternative to a numerical or written Likert scale for young children or emergent/nonreaders.

Sample questions to gain student feedback.

• This sensory tool makes me feel: better, worse, the same.
• This sensory tool helps me focus on the teacher: always, sometimes, never.
• The noise in the classroom distracts me from my work: always, sometimes, never.
• The lights in the classroom distract me from my work: always, sometimes, never.
• The classroom is just right for my learning: always, sometimes, never.
• I wish I had _____ to help me focus on my schoolwork.

Positive Behavior Interventions and Supports

School-wide sensory interventions should fall under positive behavior interventions and support (PBI&S), which is the portion of MTSS that focuses on supporting social, emotional, and behavioral (SEB) needs of students. Under a SEB MTSS framework, the goal is to prevent, teach, and respond at each tier level (Simonsen et al., 2022). Although often not thought of as part of the SEB team, the occupational therapist has much to offer in prevention, teaching, and responding under a PBI&S model. As the experts in sensory integration and processing theory, evaluation, and intervention, the occupational therapy team is the only school staff qualified to adequately address sensory needs within any frameworks. Yet, the occupational therapist is rarely part of the MTSS planning team. In many districts, interventions, such as brain breaks, which give students time to relax or break from learning, are part of the PBI&S plan. In essence, brain breaks are methods of implementing sensory strategies and supports. When the occupational therapist is involved in the planning and implementation, these breaks could meet the sensory needs of the students rather than just being a general break from learning.

In addition, as occupational therapists are experts in how clients develop and maintain routines, they are perhaps the most knowledgeable professionals in the school setting on the impact of school routines on behavior patterns. Therefore, the occupational therapist should be involved in planning and implementing PBI&S supports, such as brain breaks, so that the interventions will be more effective, tailored to the needs of the students, and performed at the best time to positively influence student performance. The occupational therapist is also an expert on the impact of the environment on participation, learning, and behavior and is best equipped to help teachers and administrators design sensory environments that are most conducive to the learning needs of the students. Finally, occupational therapists also have training in trauma-informed care and health and wellness, which is an important skill set in the PBI&S team (Center on PBI&S, 2024) and can therefore work with school personnel to develop more targeted interventions for students with histories of trauma that may have additional SEB needs.

The use of sensory interventions as part of the PBI&S plan can result in improvements in school-wide behavior. The occupational therapist may need to advocate for involvement in the PBI&S plan and implementation team, which will be discussed further in Chapter 8. However, an understanding of how sensory interventions are implemented at a Tier 1 and Tier 2 level under a PBI&S model is clear. Areas that sensory interventions may improve include the following.

- Students will listen attentively when the teacher or other students are speaking without interrupting.
- Students will arrive on time for class with all assignments and materials.
- Students will follow school rules to walk in the hallway safely and quietly.
- Students will use equipment safely and properly.
- Students will keep their hands, feet, and objects to themselves.
- Students will participate in class activities and discussions, maintaining positive interactions and attention.
- Students will work in groups and respect others, taking turns and sharing resources.
- Students will set personal goals for behavior improvement, reflect on their behavior, and work to improve it.

Progress Monitoring

Under MTSS, progress monitoring is the standard process of monitoring the effectiveness of the interventions implemented at each tiered level of support. It is evidence-based and provides a methodical process of collecting data at various points to provide a full picture of the student's performance (Clark & Miller, 1996). Progress monitoring occurs across disciplines and is standard practice in most school systems. According to the Center on Multi-Tiered System of Supports (AIR, 2024), progress monitoring is used to assess performance, quantify the progress and responsiveness of students, and evaluate effectiveness. The process involves several data collection points in a frequent and standardized manner.

The Center on Multi-Tiered System of Supports (AIR, 2024) includes a six-step process for effective progress monitoring. **Step one** is to design the process to monitor data, including frequency, format, storage, and how to analyze it. When looking at sensory-related data, the occupational therapist has the knowledge and responsibility to guide the development of this process. The occupational therapist's understanding of proximal and distal outcomes will allow for translating how sensory processing may impact the student's performance and develop effective progress monitoring processes. For example, the occupational therapist may link sensory processing needs to sustain attention or on-task behaviors as an outcome. The occupational therapist may then develop a monitoring process based on assessment of school and classroom routines.

Step two is to select the progress monitoring tools. In the case of sensory supports, the occupational therapist can efficiently utilize already established progress monitoring tools. In fact, as a related service, the occupational therapist should embed the progress monitoring within other tools the school utilizes. It is important to remember that there may be academic and/or behavioral monitoring tools that can be used to monitor the progress of the sensory interventions. If there is not one available, the occupational therapist should develop a tool to track data on provided goals in accordance with the district guidelines.

The **third step** is to train staff in monitoring progress. This training must include demonstration and checking for understanding, as it is important to ensure staff understands what behaviors they are monitoring. The occupational therapist should also ensure that staff can distinguish what should be monitored and what is not relevant. Frequency counts on designated tracking sheets are an excellent way to keep track of data. Figure 6.1 provides an example of a data sheet which can be used by occupational therapists and those who they train to monitor progress. These progress monitoring plans should also include frequency of data collection, baseline data, goals, decision rules, and dates to review data. In addition to this, fidelity to the intervention, which will be explained in detail next, should be reviewed for quality, duration, student engagement, and whether the intervention is delivered as intended (AIR, 2022).

The **final step** in the process is to analyze data to determine the effectiveness and the next course of the intervention. We will review this in the next section.

Fidelity of Interventions

Under MTSS and progress monitoring, interventions must have good fidelity, meaning they should be implemented as designed and intended according to pre-established procedures and guidelines. Measures of fidelity in MTSS include assessing the accuracy and consistency of interventions. It is an essential component because, without fidelity, data is meaningless. After all, the intended intervention is not necessarily the intervention that is being measured.

Tracking Sheet

Student's Name _____

Goals: Students will increase their time on task by 80% from the baseline.
Baseline: Averaged 5 minutes of on-task behavior before requiring assistance from school personnel to remain on task.

Criteria: Time in minutes the student engaged in academic-related tasks without prompts or assistance from the teacher.
-   The student was working on assigned work.
-   The student was at their desk or other area designated by the teacher to complete the task.
-   The student did not talk with other students unless instructed to do so.

Date/Time	Observer	Intervention Provided	Time on Task (in minutes)

Figure 6.1 Tracking sheet for monitoring progress. Image by author.

To ensure fidelity, there are many factors that need to be considered and upheld during the assessment process. Support must be provided at each tier, and the interventions must be evidence-based to reinforce the goals established by the MTSS team. Additionally, the implementation of interventions must be consistent when provided in various settings in the school, including the classroom, playground, lunchroom, hallways, etc. All staff must be on board with implementation and able to provide uniform support. Staff training is paramount in ensuring consistent, competent, and skillful implementation of interventions. Before and during the assessment process, staff may need several training sessions to ensure they fully understand what is required of them, and fidelity checks should be in place to identify if further training is needed. The relationship between staff and students is also monitored during the assessment of fidelity. Staff should ensure students stay engaged in the sensory interventions, respond positively to the interventions, and that interventions are high quality.

Finally, regular feedback from all stakeholders, including staff, parents, and students, in conjunction with regular assessment data, provides a complete picture of the effectiveness of the interventions and attitudes of reception. The occupational therapist can take these steps to ensure the fidelity of sensory interventions at all tiers and that quality data that can be used to make decisions and support positive change (Center on PBI&S, 2019).

Many districts have progress monitoring plans, so this text will not discuss the specifics of progress monitoring programs or methods. However, occupational therapists should be involved in planning and implementation, especially for fidelity checks regarding sensory interventions for progress monitoring. It is the occupational therapist's role to have frequent informal and formal check-ins with staff, ensuring that they are implementing and monitoring sensory-based interventions and sensory environmental supports correctly. The occupational therapist should also assist in data analysis and adjust interventions appropriately based on the provided data. In addition, it is essential to garner feedback from the students on the effectiveness of interventions. If the outcome is improving on-task behaviors, the questions to gain feedback from students must be about on-task behaviors, not how a particular intervention makes their body feel. Using this feedback, occupational therapists can adjust interventions as needed.

Gathering Quality Data

Quality data is essential to progress monitoring. When objectives are clearly defined and easy to measure, it is easy to gather high-quality, usable data. Quality data helps identify disparities and allows for adjustments to meet diverse needs that exist in populations and groups. It also aligns with the American occupational therapy practice framework: Domain and process–Fourth edition (OTPF-4), which indicates that individuals who are part of a group or population should be considered as individuals within the group and population and in how they interact with each other.

The first step in gathering quality data is determining the relevant metrics that will indicate how progress toward goals will be monitored. The metric should match what is being measured, and metrics should be standardized so that multiple people can gather data with comparable results. For example, if the goal is to improve time on a task from 5 minutes to 15 minutes, then the metric would be in minutes. Multiple data sources are also important, and data should be collected at various times.

Progress Monitoring Tracking Sheet

Student Name: _____   Grade: _____   Teacher: _____

		Date				
Goal	Notes					

Amount of Assistance/Prompts:
1: Continuous 90–100% of the time
2: Frequent 75% of the time
3: Occasional 50% of the time
4: Intermittent 25% of the time
5: Independent <10% of the time

Types of Assistance/Prompts
1: Physical
2: Gestural/modelling
3: Visual
4: Verbal
5: No prompt

Figure 6.2 Sample progress monitoring tracking sheet. Image by author.

There should be a plan as to how data will be gathered, stored, and tracked so any team member can add it to the full data set. Most school districts have specified methods for storing and monitoring data for progress monitoring. When working at the various tiers, the occupational therapist needs to be educated in how data is tracked and stored for the Tier 1 and Tier 2 levels, as this may differ from how Tier 3 data is stored. Figure 6.2 presents an example of a progress monitoring sheet that adheres to these criteria of collecting quality data. And, once the quality data is collected, you can begin to make decisions on what interventions to implement to help the students' sensory processing needs.

Using Data to Make Decisions on Interventions

A baseline is the solid and sound starting point that serves as the basis of comparison for progress. Baseline data is often gathered during the initial evaluation when goals are established. Once the baseline has been established, data should be gathered at regular intervals by school team members implementing the interventions. This includes the occupational therapy practitioner, other support staff, and teachers. Regardless of who is collecting the data, it is the responsibility of the occupational therapist to analyze the data to determine the success of the sensory intervention. Taking several data points in various environments and situations is important because progress can fluctuate. The goal is to identify patterns or trends in the data and make decisions based on trends rather than a single data point.

Based on the data, the occupational therapist can continue, discontinue, or modify the intervention. When the intervention is modified, adjustments are made to the original intervention. Adjustments may include the frequency of the intervention, the intensity of the intervention, or the type of intervention. For example, if providing movement breaks two times a day results in some improvements but they are inconsistent, the occupational therapist may decide to increase the frequency of movement breaks to three times per day. If that intervention is modified, new baseline data should be gathered to determine if the modification has been successful. The information gathered during progress monitoring can also be used to determine the need for additional supports or a change in tier level of services. When a goal is modified or a new goal is generated, a new baseline should be established.

Using Data to Make Treatment Decisions

When an intervention is implemented with good fidelity and targeted at the area of need, the occupational therapist should expect progress, even if it is slow. When progress does not occur as expected, the occupational therapist must examine the intervention to determine what, if anything, needs to be changed. Many areas may need to be modified.

- **Fidelity of implementation**: The occupational therapist must determine if the interventions are being performed as intended. If the therapist is not performing the intervention, they should observe it. If the intervention is not being performed correctly, the occupational therapist should retrain the person implementing it, providing additional instruction and opportunities for teach-back and demonstration. They should also ensure the person is competent and understands the intervention before performing it with a student.
  - **Solution**: Retrain and complete frequent fidelity checks.
- **Frequency of implementation**: The frequency at which the intervention is performed may need to be adjusted. This process can use trial and error to determine the best frequency for any particular intervention. During this process, data will be gathered either more or less frequently to determine if changes in intervention frequency impact outcomes.
  - **Solution**: Change the frequency of intervention and collect frequent data to determine the optimal frequency.

- **Type of intervention/frame of reference**: In some circumstances, the intervention is not the best for the student, or the frame of reference for treatment is not what the student needs. When the intervention has been implemented with good fidelity over time but does not demonstrate progress, the occupational therapist may need to take another look at the underlying issues that may be causing participation barriers. A new issue may have arisen, or something may have been misidentified in the evaluation process. Evaluation data will help determine if a new type of intervention needs to be implemented.
    - **Solution**: Perform formal or informal evaluation to determine if new or different needs are identified. Change the plan of care if needed.
- **Environment**: The environment may be hindering the student's progress. This is often determined if the student does well in one environment and not in another. If that is the case, the occupational therapist may not need to modify the intervention. Rather, they may need to address a specific environment.
    - **Solution**: Modify the environment where the student is having difficulty.
- **Method of intervention**: There are times when the intervention is performed with good fidelity, at a good frequency, and is the best type of intervention, but it is ineffective when implemented by certain individuals. While some people may do interventions correctly, they lack a connection with the student. In occupational therapy, this is known as therapeutic use of self. Sometimes there is a mismatch between the person and the client due to something beyond the control of anyone, such as personality. In this case, finding a new person to implement the intervention may be best.
    - **Solution**: Find a new person to implement the intervention that may have a better match with the students.

Once the progress data is gathered, the occupational therapist and the MTSS team can easily see trends. If the trends do not indicate improvement, the occupational therapist and MTSS team must engage in the problem-solving process to determine the reason for the lack of progress. When a solution is implemented, the frequency of data collection should increase to evaluate its effectiveness.

When examining the effectiveness of interventions, the occupational therapist needs to address other barriers that may hinder the client's progress. These barriers may be environmental, attitudinal, or personal, and they may also be related to other factors outside the school setting. The occupational therapist can review and address potential barriers in the modified intervention. All intervention modifications should be documented and communicated with team members, including the student and parents. As addressed in Chapter 2, open communication with everyone involved is key to ensuring the success of the implementation of interventions and to addressing potential barriers.

However, if a client responds positively to interventions, the occupational therapist can begin to look at discharge planning.

Discharge Planning

As the goal of occupational therapy is to facilitate occupational adaptation, the occupational therapist should consider discharge planning as soon as the client initiates occupational therapy services. Occupational adaptation involves the client responding to occupational and contextual demands efficiently and effectively (Grajo, 2019). When the occupational therapist chooses which assessment methods to initiate the occupational therapy process, consideration of repeated outcomes to determine the need for discharge is part of the decision-making process. Using the same outcomes can help determine if there is an ongoing need for occupational therapy services or if services should be transitioned to different levels of support or discontinued altogether. Discontinuation of services is often considered when the client has met their goals and reached a point where they can successfully manage their needs with sustainability plans to ensure their long-term success (AOTA, 2020). Discharge planning varies depending on whether the client is in Tier 1, 2, or 3, so these approaches need to be considered independently.

Discharge Planning for Tier 1

Sustainability plans for groups and populations provide strategies to help ensure a program's continued success without direct support. Therefore, the occupational therapist can help ensure resources are available to help adapt to the changing circumstances, while continuing the sensory programs provided at the group and population levels. The occupational therapist should continue building capacity for the program through staff training and professional development, and they also should be involved in program evaluation to meet the needs of the group or population. Establishing networks of teachers and support personnel to problem solve and brainstorm additional methods of sensory input within the school setting is vital to ongoing success. As occupational therapists ensure sustainability, they can provide less direct support, especially at the population level. However, the occupational therapist should continue to be involved throughout the process and increase support as needed.

Discharge Planning for Tier 2 and Tier 3

Often, discharge planning involves a transition of services. This is especially true when working under an MTSS model. Students may move up or down tiers, which provide more or less support, depending on their needs. This is known as transition planning and requires preparation guided by the occupational therapist. All parties, including teachers, school support staff, parents, and students, must be aware of the transition process. One benefit of the occupational therapist being involved in each tier of support is that all students receive sensory supports from the occupational therapist, whether receiving special education services, Response to Intervention (RTI), or general education.

When occupational therapists are involved at each level of MTSS, a transition between tiers is much easier and more fluid.

Many parents may become nervous when children no longer need Tier 3 services. This is understandable as often, before receiving individualized education program (IEP) services, their child may have been struggling with many aspects of the school day. Now that the child is doing well, the parents may be concerned that pulling back support will cause their child to struggle again. If the school promotes occupational therapy being involved at Tier 1 and Tier 2 levels, then the child can simply move down a level of support. Remember, students receiving higher levels of support (i.e. Tier 3) are still provided support at lower-tiered levels. Under the MTSS model, the occupational therapist still monitors the student and tailors interventions as needed, just under a different tier level. While direct services under an IEP may be discharged, the student can still access services via MTSS and receive support with less direct and targeted intervention. When parents understand that their child will still receive some level of support, this can help ease their minds about transitioning away from the IEP and special education services.

Consultation Services

Occupational therapists may provide services via consultation. This frequently occurs as part of the transition plan when a child begins to move out of a Tier 3 level of support. With consultation, the occupational therapist provides support, advice, and guidance on a specific area of need. In the school setting, consultation usually occurs with the teacher, to provide suggestions and strategies to assist the child in particular areas. Consultation is a service delivery model, so the occupational therapy process should still be followed, beginning with assessment. Goals may focus more on independence in the classroom or how the teacher can support the child in the classroom. Self-advocacy goals are excellent for the consultation model of service as they promote independence toward the transition of services.

Let us see how this all comes together in practice through a case example, following Anabelle's experience of evaluation, implementation, progress monitoring, and transitioning between occupational therapy services and tiers in Box 6.1.

BOX 6.1   CASE EXAMPLE

Anabelle received a diagnosis of autism spectrum disorder when she was six years old. During first grade, she struggled in the classroom with following routines, staying on task, and interacting with others. She had frequent referrals for behaviors such as hitting and biting. She also struggled academically with reading and writing. She was identified through universal screening as needing additional behavioral and academic support and received services through RTI.

However, as the school year progressed, Anabelle continued to struggle. Eventually, a special education referral was made. Anabelle was evaluated, and the team determined that she met the criteria for special education under the eligibility category of autism. Anabelle received specialized instruction, behavioral support, occupational therapy, and speech-language therapy. With this level of support, she was much more successful in her second and third grade years.

She continued to make progress and required less direct support. By her fourth grade year, the occupational therapist structured Anabelle's day so that she could participate in the small sensory group the occupational therapy assistant ran three times a week. Anabelle enjoyed this group and was able to begin to advocate for her own sensory needs in this small group setting. In addition, the occupational therapist checked in frequently with the classroom teacher to ensure Anabelle could access activities and equipment to meet her sensory needs. She helped the teacher problem-solve any areas of difficulty and provided additional recommendations as warranted. Eventually, the IEP team determined that Anabelle no longer needed direct occupational therapy services.

When this information was presented to the parents, the occupational therapist showed them that Anabelle could still access sensory supports, participate in a small group focused on sensory processing needs, and access sensory tools in the classroom. Furthermore, the classroom teacher implemented the *Zones of Regulation* program to help all students monitor and meet their sensory needs. Anabelle had been working on this program in occupational therapy as well and could utilize the tools across settings. The parents were happy to hear that Anabelle could spend more time in the classroom focusing on academic tasks and still have a level of support for her sensory needs.

Summary

In this chapter we explored the importance of outcomes for making decisions regarding sensory interventions. Occupational therapists use a variety of outcome measures, standardized and unstandardized, formal and informal, to measure progress and make decisions about interventions. Therefore, it is important for occupational therapists to understand quality outcomes, including psychometric properties and the intent of the outcomes. Understanding the psychometric properties of formal assessments can help the occupational therapist choose the best outcome measure for the client at all MTSS levels.

This chapter then explored the importance of working with the MTSS planning team to be integrally involved with the universal screening, progress monitoring, and PBI&S planning. The occupational therapist has expert training in sensory integration theory, assessment, and intervention and should be involved with the MTSS planning team to ensure that sensory integration and processing is considered at all MTSS levels when evaluating outcomes.

The chapter concluded with a discussion on how to ensure data is of high quality and how to use data to make decisions about what step to take next. In addition, we discussed the importance of discharge considerations throughout the occupational therapist and how discharge planning may look at each of the tier levels.

In Chapter 7 we will discuss the importance of working with a multidisciplinary team to ensure that sensory interventions are implemented in the best way possible to support students at all MTSS levels.

References

American Institutes for Research (AIR) (2024). *Center on multi-tiered systems of support: Progress monitoring.* https://mtss4success.org/essential-components/progress-monitoring.

American Institutes for Research (AIR) (2022, October 28). *MTSS infrastructure and support mechanisms series.* https://mtss4success.org.

American Occupational Therapy Association (AOTA) (2020). Occupational therapy practice framework: Domain and process–Fourth edition (OTPF-4). *American Journal of Occupational Therapy, 74*(S2), 1–85. https://doi.org/10.5014/ajot.2020.74S2001.

Badrick, T. & Bowling, F. (2023). Clinical utility-information about the usefulness of tests. *Clinical Biochemistry*, 110656. https://doi.org.10.1016/j.clinbiochem.2023.110656.

Blanche, E. I., Reinoso, G., & Kiefer, D. B. (2021). *Structured Observations of Sensory Integration- Motor (SOSI-M).* ATP Assessments.

Bowyer, P., Kramer, J., Ploszaj, A., Ross, M., Schwartz, O., Kielhofner, G., & Kramer, K. (2008). *A users manual for the Short Child Occupational Profile (SCOPE) [Version 2.2.].* The Model of Human Occupation Clearinghouse. Department of Occupational Therapy. University of Illinois at Chicago

Center on Positive Behavioral Interventions & Supports (PBI&S) (2019, April 1). *PBIS Tiered Fidelity Inventory*. https://www.pbis.org/resource/tfi.

Center on Positive Behavioral Interventions & Supports (PBI&S) (2024). *Tier 1*. https://www.pbis.org/pbis/tier-1.

Clark, G. F. & Miller, L. E. (1996). Providing effective occupational therapy services: Data-based decision making in school-based practice. *American Journal of Occupational Therapy*, *50*(9), 701–708. https://doi.org/10.5014/ajot.50.9.701.

Dunn, W. (2014). *Sensory Profile 2*. Pearson Assessments.

Grajo, L. (2019). Theory of occupational adaptation. In B. A. B. Schell & G. Gillen (eds), *Willard and Spackman's Occupational Therapy*, 13th ed., pp. 633–642. Wolters Kluwer.

Griswold, L. A. (2014). Evaluation in the intervention planning process. In J. Hinojosa & P. Kramer (eds), *Evaluation in Occupational Therapy: Obtaining and Interpreting Data*, 4th ed., pp. 65–86. AOTA Press.

Mailloux, Z., Parham, L.D., Roley, S. S., Ruzzano, L., & Schaaf, R. C. (2018). Introduction to the Evaluation in Ayres Sensory Integration®(EASI). *American Journal of Occupational Therapy, 72*, 7201195030p1–7201195030p7. https://doi.org/10.5014/ajot.2018.028241.

Miller, L. J., Oakland, T., Herzber, D. S. (2013). *Goal Oriented Assessment of Lifeskills (GOAL™)*. Western Psychological Services.

Missall, K., Artman-Meeker, K., Roberts, C., & Ludeman, S. (2021). Implementing multitiered systems of support in preschool: Begin with universal screening. *Young Exceptional Children*, *24*(4), 213–224. https://doi.org/10.1177/1096250620931807.

Parham, L. D., Ecker, C. L., Kuhaneck, H., Henry, D. A., & Glennon, T. J. (2021). *Sensory Processing Measure, Second Edition (SPM-2)*. Western Psychological Services.

Portney, L. G. (2020). *Foundations of Clinical Research: Application to Evidence-Based Practice* (4th ed.). F. A. Davis.

Schell, B. A. B. & Gillen, G. (2019). Glossary. In B.A.B. Schell & G. Gillen (eds), *Willard and Spackman's Occupational Therapy,* 13th ed. Wolters Kluwer.

Simonsen, B., Robbie, K., Meyer, K., Freeman, J., Everett, S., & Feinberg, A. B. (2022). Supporting students' social, emotional, and behavior (SEB) growth through Tier 2 and 3 intervention within a multi-tiered system of supports (MTSS) framework. In E. J. Sabornie & D. L. Espelage (eds), *Handbook of Classroom Management*, 3rd ed., pp. 102–127. Routledge.

Stansberry, A. & Piller, A. (2023). *The Sensory and Satisfaction Questionnaire* [Unpublished Assessment].

Chapter 7

Working with a Multidisciplinary Team

Introduction

When working to support students and their sensory needs, it is crucial to recognize that it takes a village. If a person is removed from the support network, the whole school setting is impacted – most significantly, the students with access needs. As school budgets are constantly under threat of being reduced, school personnel are under pressure to prove the value of key roles, such as occupational therapists, at varying tier levels.

This chapter discusses the increasing need for sensory support for students of all ages and how administrators and teachers can advocate for an increased occupational therapist role at all MTSS levels. It highlights the benefits of an occupational therapist working at the lower tier levels, including lowering costs, decreasing burnout, providing support for teaching staff, and improving implementation with federal requirements. It will then discuss how occupational therapists can work within the multidisciplinary team of the school setting with a particular focus on training teachers and classroom assistants to implement interventions with good fidelity.

Increased Need for Sensory Support

In today's educational system, students are diverse with varying needs and learning styles. As a result, there is undoubtedly an increased need for sensory support. The prevalence of sensory processing differences continues to increase (Ben-Sasson et al., 2009; Jussila et al., 2020) and there is also an increased awareness of how sensory processing impacts student performance. However, due to contemporary technological advances and our growing reliance on this technology, many children have decreased opportunities for free play and engagement in unstructured gross motor activities, both in and outside the school environment. As discussed in Chapter 6, free play provides opportunities for children to meet many different sensory needs in a way that is best for their bodies and minds, and without this, children do not gain the sensory input they need to

DOI: 10.4324/9781032654768-8

regulate and perform their daily activities at the most optimal level. Educators strive to support all students within the structure of the mainstream classroom through universal design for learning, and occupational therapists who work within a tiered system have the opportunity to impact many students and school staff across the entire school population, and even the district. As a result, many students in the general education classroom can benefit from sensory support to facilitate learning and positive behavior.

Despite this need for increased sensory supports school-wide, many school personnel, administrators, and staff may initially be reluctant to consider implementing additional support. They may be afraid that adding one more activity to their day will overwhelm them and their students as the demands for instructional time and support continually increase. Many school districts may view an additional implementation of supports under the multi-tiered systems of supports (MTSS) model as more work for teachers and assistants. However, the MTSS model is designed to help alleviate the burden on school personnel by providing interventions before students require more intensified support, which would require additional time, staff, and resources. If implemented in a specified manner, providing sensory supports can significantly reduce the teachers' burden by increasing student engagement, participation, and attention to academic tasks, decreasing maladaptive and off-task behaviors. In addition, under the MTSS model, the occupational therapy team can dedicate time to training and assisting teachers and classroom assistants to provide the most effective sensory supports embedded in the classroom routine and school day. As a result, improvements in classroom performance should be seen immediately.

Many sensory supports are easy to implement, and their positive results extend beyond the classroom setting (Bodison & Parham, 2018). Occupational therapists often exist in the background of the school setting, servicing clients through the special education department under individualized education programs (IEPs). As a result, mainstream administrators and teachers in general education may have limited exposure to the occupational therapy team and minimal understanding of the scope and breadth of occupational therapy's role in the school. They may need help understanding how much information and support the occupational therapy practitioner can provide in the general education setting and under MTSS. It is the responsibility of the occupational therapy team to help school personnel and administrators understand the value of occupational therapy. The occupational therapist themselves must become their own promoter and work to demonstrate the value of occupational therapy interventions performed at various tiered levels. While this may seem staggering to the occupational therapist at first, it will create improved collaboration and decrease the burden of direct treatment for therapists who are already overworked in understaffed therapy teams. In addition, it will ease the workload of the teacher and improve student performance.

When occupational therapy practitioners work at all MTSS levels, there is an opportunity for collaboration and interprofessional support. However, occupational therapy practitioners face many challenges in becoming more involved in the Tier 1 and Tier 2 levels. First, many occupational therapy practitioners are contract employees of the school rather than being employed by the school district. When schools hire contractors to provide therapy services, their contracts are often developed based on the number of service minutes students have in their IEPs. The service minutes are used to determine the number of hours or number of therapists the school needs to fulfill these minutes. Therefore, therapy personnel are expected to spend most of their paid contracted time fulfilling these minutes. This caseload model focuses on ensuring students are served for their IEP minutes, and occupational therapy practitioners must maintain high levels of billable time during their workday. Being expected to spend most of their time delivering therapy services in fulfillment of IEP requirements can make implementing services at any level other than a Tier 3 difficult.

The medical model of occupational therapy continues to dominate the structure of occupational therapy practice, even in the school system. This causes practitioners and administrators to see occupational therapy as only servicing students at the Tier 3 level via an individualized service model. Also, since occupational therapy practitioners are commonly employed through outside agencies, often they are not viewed as part of the school team. As a result, occupational therapy practitioners need to take the lead on advocating for this change. It is much more natural to be seen as a part of the school team when the occupational therapy practitioner is a school employee. In addition to this, being a school employee has multiple benefits. It affords the opportunity for the occupational therapy practitioner to be compensated for time spent in meetings, training, and supporting teachers and students at lower MTSS levels, rather than only for direct services in Tier 3. As well as this, being a school employee can allow occupational therapy practitioners to receive some of the benefits of being state employees, including retirement, that may help compensate for a lower pay rate than a contractor rate.

While it is ideal for the occupational therapy practitioner to be a school employee, being a school contractor does not prevent the occupational therapy practitioner from being a school team member. However, it does shift more of the responsibility onto the therapist to promote themselves as being an integral part of the team. Consequently, the occupational therapist may need to offer their time and dedication outside of paid hours. Being a part of staff and department meetings, even if not paid, can go a long way in being seen as a team member. Also, performing training at professional development days provides an opportunity for many staff members to get to know the occupational therapy team and see the value they bring to the school setting beyond just servicing students on their IEP. Attending meetings and other school events, even if not required, can lay the foundation for building relationships, making lasting changes in how the occupational therapy practitioner works with the team.

From this, what is clear is that a shift in thinking is needed in the field. Let us review the benefits of moving from a caseload to workload model before understanding how we can promote this change to school personnel.

Shift in Thinking

Occupational therapy services in the school setting traditionally follow a caseload model. Many school administrators, teachers, and parents expect this service delivery model when a student receives occupational therapy services in an IEP or 504 plan. However, given the current needs, especially those related to sensory processing, occupational therapy is primed for a different model of practice that extends beyond the one-on-one or small-group treatment model. Although paradigm shifts are often met with resistance, this shift is necessary in order to best support students at all tier levels in the educational setting.

Thomas Kuhn wrote about the concept of "paradigm shift" in his 1962 book *The Structure of Scientific Revolutions.* Since then, the term "paradigm shift" has become familiar with seismic, rather than gradual, changes in traditional thinking. In today's educational system, teachers are constantly asked to implement new or different programs, change their education model, and accommodate learners' diverse needs. Many educators are exhausted by these changes, face burnout, and feel overwhelmed by the idea of learning and implementing a new model (Lillard, 2023). Occupational therapy practitioners in the school setting face demands similar to those of teachers, with high caseloads, increased referrals, and increased requirements for paperwork, all while facing a shortage of available therapists. While the idea of implementing a new philosophy of service delivery may seem daunting, according to Kuhn, the stressors of the current climate present the perfect opportunity for a paradigm shift. The present model of occupational therapy services in the school system does not provide the most effective care to students and is not the most efficient use of the occupational therapy team's time and resources. More and more students face an increased need for sensory input and behavioral support using sensory strategies. These needs can easily result in poor academic performance for students who struggle with paying attention, following directions, comprehending directions, and completing assignments, all signs frequently seen in children with sensory processing differences. Unmet sensory needs can also result in behavioral difficulties such as off-task behaviors, refusals to participate in classroom tasks and activities, and even aggressive behaviors towards other students and staff. If a student's sensory needs were met, the result would be increased academic achievement, improved behavior (Ayres, 1979), and decreased referrals for special education services that require high levels of support and resources in an already strained system. Therefore, the time for a paradigm shift is now.

The Shift from Caseload to Workload

For this shift to happen in school settings, the main change required is for occupational therapists to move from a caseload to workload model. The caseload approach is rooted in the traditional medical model of treating patients one-on-one, working on goals designed explicitly in a plan of care. A caseload consists of a number of clients the occupational therapy practitioner is responsible for providing treatment for over a specific period and for a set amount of time. In the school setting, it is often referred to as one of two things: the number of students or the number of service minutes one therapist is responsible for providing. Students are scheduled for occupational therapy and seen during their scheduled time, just as they would be in an outpatient therapy medical practice. This includes students with regular weekly or monthly minutes on an IEP and those with consultative minutes.

Overall, a caseload represents the work and responsibilities of the occupational therapy practitioner to provide support to students, teachers, and support staff. However, the therapists' schedules are often full of service minutes from the start to the end of the day, leaving little time for other responsibilities. The occupational therapy practitioner has to balance competing priorities and allocate resources while providing quality services to the students for the designated amount of time outlined by the IEP. They have minimal, if any, time for other activities, including collaboration with other school personnel. Therefore, they are frequently not seen as part of the more comprehensive education team outside of special education. They may be undervalued by school personnel, administrators, or parents because they have no time to build relationships and offer additional services to the school (Rioux & Jackson, 2019). Given the increased sensory processing needs of students and the importance of promoting good mental health, the caseload model is not necessarily the best use of the occupational therapy practitioner's time.

In contrast, the workload approach to occupational therapy differs in structure and philosophy. The workload approach looks at the therapist's responsibilities as a whole rather than focusing only on the service minutes. The number of students and service minutes are considered part of the therapy caseload, but many other aspects are considered when using a workload model. This includes direct services, indirect services, administrative work, paperwork, other compliance work, and other daily activities such as travel time and professional training (American Speech-Language-Hearing Association, 2024; Rioux & Jackson, 2019). Therapists engage in many activities during the day but may only document their time spent in direct service with students, as district and regulatory policies and best practice guidelines require. However, occupational therapy practitioners should be in the habit of documenting all activities they perform during their working hours, whether they are spent in direct service of students or in related activities. This allows the therapist and administration to see that other responsibilities go into servicing the students and provides a log of all the requirements for successfully implementing occupational therapy services in the school setting. In addition, it helps the occupational therapy practitioner know where there is time to spend on additional activities, such as training staff and servicing all students through MTSS levels.

The workload model allows the occupational therapy practitioner to use time in various ways to service clients without a service minutes mindset. The occupational therapy practitioner can provide services in the classroom setting in collaboration with teachers, provide interdisciplinary services, and even service students in settings where they may need support, such as physical education classes or the cafeteria. This allows services to be given to individuals who may receive direct service minutes and those not on caseload. In addition to this, the workload model is a team approach – several school personnel work together to provide holistic support to individual students, groups of students, classroom activities, and school-wide activities. It allows for increased daily time for direct service personnel, such as occupational therapists and speech-language pathologists, to service more clients and provide better support for school staff (Seruya & Garfinkel, 2020). As the occupational therapist works as a team with other school personnel, such as teachers, it is a more efficient way of managing required tasks across multiple people, promoting balance across the team rather than overloading one individual. As there is increased transparency and clear allocation of roles, it also encourages teamwork and accountability while working toward the IEP goals. The approach is also flexible to change based on the needs, priorities, and available resources. Overall, workload approaches lead to improved employee satisfaction, better distribution of work, and decreased burnout among therapists.

Moving from a caseload to a workload model requires organizational change for districts to embed occupational therapy in the Tier 1 and Tier 2 levels. It is the occupational therapist's role to promote this change, and it is important to review how they can gather this organizational support

Gathering Organizational Support

If the occupational therapy team is going to make changes to the structure and organization of the school, they must advocate for the support of the administration. Working with leadership to demonstrate the value of change is essential, but it can also be intimidating. By following a systematic approach and presenting supporting data, the occupational therapy team can increase their chances of the administration accepting a change in attitude, views, and organization (Cornelius & Gustafson, 2020).

The occupational therapist must gain administrative and teacher support to implement a successful sensory program at Tier 1 and Tier 2 levels. To achieve this, two main points need to be developed to lay the foundation for gathering organizational support. The main concerns for administrators are the workings of their schools and districts and ensuring that their staff have the support and resources they need to be successful, all while being mindful of budgets and staffing. Therefore, when presenting a change in model from implementing occupational therapy services at only Tier 3 to also including them at Tier 1 and Tier 2, the occupational therapy team must stress how implementation at these levels can save the school time and money.

Schools are typically reimbursed through the state Medicaid program for direct occupational therapy services provided to students under an IEP. Administrators may initially be hesitant to provide occupational therapy practitioners time to engage in other activities outside of direct, billable treatment time, as this is a source of revenue to pay the salaries of occupational therapy practitioners, who tend to be higher-paid school employees. Providing information on how implementing services at Tier 1 and Tier 2 levels can save significant staff and monetary resources can help administrators see past the initial request of allowing occupational therapy practitioners to engage in services that may not be billable to Medicaid. Next, teachers must see occupational therapy practitioners as a support to their needs as classroom teachers. By forming a collaborative relationship and focusing on the teachers' needs, rather than being a staff member who provides even more suggestions on how to modify instruction, the occupational therapy practitioner can be seen as an ally. When occupational therapists work with teachers to support classroom needs, teachers see them as assets. The teachers can provide positive feedback to the administration regarding the impact of the occupational therapy department. With this in mind, let us take a look at how occupational therapists can practically advocate for their roles in Tier 1 and Tier 2.

How to Advocate for Time in Tier 1 and Tier 2

It can be daunting for occupational therapy practitioners to approach school administrators for more time providing services at Tier 1 and Tier 2 levels. However, the most effective way to approach this is by presenting the benefits of incorporating the occupational therapy team into Tier 1 and Tier 2 interventions. These benefits include cost savings, improved academic performance, and decreased behavioral referrals. One way this can be shown is by sharing the results of the progress monitoring process, as this data can demonstrate the value of occupational therapy practitioners intervening at lower tiers. Nonetheless, occupational therapy practitioners are often already busy with providing services to students receiving special education, and they may need more time and resources to gather this data at Tiers 1 and 2. The goal is that by initially providing additional resources, the school can shift to support more students with occupational therapy at lower tier levels, thus preventing many students from needing more intensified one-on-one occupational therapy services. This will save the district time, money, and resources in the long run.

To help occupational therapists pitch for this support, we will now look at what practical steps to take when approaching administrators and how to formulate a proposal for implementing interventions at Tiers 1 and 2. We will then turn to how to manage transformational change in the school setting.

Steps to Advocate for Time and Resources to Implement Tier 1 and Tier 2 Interventions

1. **Set up an appointment to meet with school administrators**
    The first step in advocating for time and resources is to set up an appointment with the school administrators, who can make decisions on the pay and structure of school personnel. This may be the school principal, special education director, or another school administrator.
2. **Clearly define and communicate the purpose of the meeting with the school administrator**
    Be sure to clearly define the objectives of the meeting. It is best to write these down and you may even want to share them with the administrator prior to the meeting. The objective may be as simple as the following:

    > *The purpose of this meeting is to discuss how the occupational therapy team can support students at all MTSS levels and help provide positive behavioral support, academic support, and decrease referrals for special education.*

    Be open and explicit about the context and purpose of your meeting. Let them know you are there to discuss how occupational therapy can benefit students and school staff and make better use of resources. Make sure they know the purpose of the meeting is to discuss what is going well with occupational therapy and how occupational therapy can further be utilized to benefit students and staff beyond how it is currently being used (Tier 3). If it is an initial meeting, the goal may just be to explore the idea of having occupational therapy involved in the MTSS planning meetings. If it is a subsequent meeting, the goal may be to begin to discuss logistics of how to implement occupational therapy at Tier 1 and Tier 2 levels.
3. **Present data to support the need for increased services and show the impact of providing services at lower Tier levels**
    Administrators need as much data as possible to support their request for additional time or resources for the Tier 1 and Tier 2 level interventions. Data should be gathered ahead of time from a variety of sources. Data can come from progress monitoring data, surveys of teachers, or qualitative reports from teachers regarding the value of occupational therapy interventions at the lower Tier levels. The occupational therapist should take time before the meeting to distribute surveys and conduct interviews to have quality data to present at the meeting.

4. **Present the proposal**

    The occupational therapy practitioner needs to develop a proposal outlining their goals, the amount of time they need, the implementation plan, and expected outcomes. They should also focus on the potential benefits, such as how students will be supported to achieve better, teachers will be assisted, and the district can save money and resources. Box 7.1 below provides a sample proposal plan that occupational therapy practitioners can modify to present to administration staff. Be sure to include summations of published research that shows the benefits of occupational therapy. The American Occupational Therapy Association (AOTA) provides many ready-made handouts that summarize the benefits of occupational therapy in the school setting and at all MTSS levels. The resources can be provided to administrators to support your proposal.

5. **Answer any questions**

    When presenting the proposal to administrators, the occupational therapy practitioner should communicate effectively and be prepared for questions. Refrain from assuming administrators know what occupational therapists do or their full scope of practice. Instead, describe the occupational therapy team's scope of practice and expertise; be specific about how occupational therapy can support sensory and behavioral needs, paving the way for improved academic achievement. Help the administration understand how sensory interventions provide an effective method of positive behavioral support.

6. **Follow up after the meeting to answer questions and address next steps**

    Follow up after the meeting to answer any additional questions and to see if the administration is ready to embark on the next steps or needs more information and time. In addition, if there are teachers who can also provide support for advocating for occupational therapy services at a lower tier, having them follow up with the administrators to provide feedback on their support can be very helpful.

BOX 7.1   SAMPLE PROPOSAL

Impact: Provide the occupational therapy team time and opportunity to provide intervention at the Tier 1 and Tier 2 levels.

Goals:

1) Provide skilled sensory supports for students, which will increase their ability to engage in academic tasks while reducing the burden to the teacher of managing off-task behaviors and reducing behavioral referrals.

2) Provide skilled sensory supports for students with more identified needs to reduce the number of students requiring more direct, intensified occupational therapy services at the Tier 3 level under an IEP.

Objectives:

1) After the implementation of occupational therapy services at the Tier 1 level, behavioral referrals will reduce by at least 30% within 90 days.
2) After occupational therapy services are implemented at the Tier 2 level, the number of occupational therapy referrals will decrease by 50% within one school year.

Plan:

- Provide school-wide training on professional development day to provide teachers and classroom assistants with information on identifying sensory needs and how to provide sensory supports within the regular routines of the classroom and school.
- Participate in the universal screening process.
- Provide sensory supports in the classroom that all students can access but may be targeted at specific needs identified through the universal screening process.
- Provide sensory support during other Response to Interventions (RTI) to assist Tier 2 groups that have been identified as having difficulty with on-task behaviors.
- Train school personnel who provide RTI on how to incorporate sensory supports into their interventions. Once trained, the occupational therapist will only need to check in rather than provide direct interventions.

Needs:

Anticipated Need	Anticipated Resources
Time for developing a professional development course	2 hours to develop 2 hours to present
Time to participate in universal screenings	1–2 days, 2–4 times a year during the universal screening process to screen classrooms
Time to design supports and collaborate with teachers to set up sensory supportive classroom environments	1–2 hours per week

Anticipated Need	Anticipated Resources
Budget for sensory tools	Variant
	Can solicit parent-teacher organization (PTO) for funds
	May use classroom budget for tools
Time to train RTI staff	1–2 hours per quarter

Timeline:

First quarter

- Provide professional development at the beginning of the year.
- Assist in universal screenings.
- Provide support for teachers to set up classrooms that offer sensory spaces and sensory opportunities.

Second quarter

- Provide additional support based on universal screening data.
- Provide training to RTI staff.

Third quarter

- Provide check-in with teachers and RTI staff for additional needs and training.
- Provide universal screening to determine the effectiveness of interventions and additional student needs.

Fourth quarter

- Report data to administration.
- Prepare training materials for next school year.

Anticipated benefits:

- Decreased burden on teachers to develop and implement sensory support plans.
- Skilled sensory supports are more effective than general sensory supports that may be ineffective.
- Improved student engagement and participation in classroom activities.
- Decreased number of referrals to occupational therapy. This can result in decreased costs to the district and balances the cost of time allowed for the occupational therapist to participate in recommended activities.

Being mindful about how and when to communicate the value of occupational therapy to other school personnel is essential to success in promoting a change of mindset. The occupational therapy team should begin with a careful and planned conversation with key stakeholders who have the ability to implement change. Here are additional tips to consider when facilitating a conversation about using occupational therapy in Tier 1 and Tier 2.

1) **Find a place where you feel comfortable talking with teachers and administrators**. It may be best to schedule time with administrators. They often have many meetings and responsibilities, so scheduling in advance allows adequate time to present the information on the benefits of workload versus caseload and how occupational therapy can improve student performance if implemented at all tier levels under MTSS. When speaking with teachers, ensure it is during their availability, such as their planning time.

2) **Be positive and respectful**. Start with positives about the current model of occupational therapy implementing services at Tier 3. Offering compliments specific to the program and the person you are talking to can help set the tone for the conversation. This can also be a good starting point to gain common ground. If all parties are in agreement on the benefits of occupational therapy services at Tier 3, they may be open to see the benefits of occupational therapy in other areas as well.

3) **Encourage reflection and feedback, and engage in active listening**. Facilitate open and respectful dialogue with honest feedback and promote brainstorming of ideas for implementation. Understand that it may take multiple meetings for other team members to be open to the idea.

4) **Ensure commitment and follow-up**. Commit to the next steps. Even if the next step is just to follow up, ensure there is a clear next step. Follow up after the meeting to thank the person for their time, remind them of the next steps, and express your excitement for the future. Let the person know you will be following up and make sure to follow up with a recap of the meeting and next steps. If another meeting is warranted, attempt to set that up when you follow up with staff or administrators. It can take several meetings, so stay diligent and do not be afraid to follow up several times, even if you do not receive a response.

By following these steps, it can help the occupational therapist start the conversation mindfully and respectfully, promoting and managing transformational change. We will now see how this can be done successfully in the school environment.

Managing Transformational Change

Knoster's Model for Managing Complex Change (1991) is a model that can be applied to help change organizational vision and gain organizational support, which can be incredibly beneficial for occupational therapists looking to extend their services to Tier 1 and 2 levels in school settings.

The first stage of the five-stage model is to help the district or school recognize a need for change. In order to help the district recognize this, the occupational therapy team needs to understand why the school operates as it does at the current time, and if the school administrators and teachers feel there is a need for change. At this stage, occupational therapy practitioners can help determine where teachers and support personnel have needs and how to address them, such as through targeted strategies to help students with behavioral difficulties, plans for improving academic performance, or resources to help students who need additional support. The occupational therapy practitioner can then take time to engage with the staff to learn their needs and work to provide direct support at that moment. This creates organizational buy-in by demonstrating how occupational therapy directly supports current needs.

Educators know that many students have sensory processing needs. This can be a great starting point for helping teachers and administrators understand there is a need for change in the role of the occupational therapy department. Since occupational therapy practitioners are experts in sensory processing, they can provide skilled recommendations to support students in their sensory processing to improve academic performance and support positive behavior interventions.

The next phase is implementation. One of the most critical aspects of change is ensuring those involved feel equipped and empowered to implement the change. The occupational therapy practitioner has a vital role in this phase. They are responsible for training staff on sensory processing, sensory needs, the impact of sensory processing on learning, and how and why to implement sensory strategies. A sample training for teachers and classroom aides should be provided, and this training can be used at an in-service or professional development day. By providing this training, it can help school staff understand the role of sensory processing and sensory supports, how to implement sensory supports, and how to work collaboratively with occupational therapy practitioners to ensure students' needs are met.

The subsequent three phases of Knoster's model are different stages of refreeze. The first phase of refreezing involves the change being embedded within the framework of the school or district. The importance of this phase is to ensure the change is sustainable within the school and, therefore, becomes permanent. The occupational therapy practitioner must monitor this change and help provide support throughout this stage. The next refreeze stage, which reviews and monitors what has been implemented, is when the occupational therapy practitioner works with staff to make necessary adjustments to ensure sustainability. They take a step back and monitor the supports in place to see if they are effective, if more supports are needed, or if the staff is moving towards independence and sustainability. The final refreeze stage embeds the change within the entire school or district's culture, which is expected and routine. This is where changes become policies and expectations of all individuals within the organization. This phase can take time, but once it becomes part of the school culture, the staff support one another to create lasting change.

Flexibility, collaboration, and communication are essential parts of Knoster's model. While many school administrators are familiar with this model, occupational therapists need to initiate their involvement. It is essential for occupational therapy practitioners to work on the art of "being at the table"; and due to administrators not understanding the positive impact and power of the occupational therapist's role on academic and behavior support, they need to promote this. Today, many entry-level occupational therapy degrees are doctoral degrees, putting occupational therapists on par with the education level of school administrators. They are well-versed in research, research strategies, and implementation of research findings. Presenting evidence-based information brings credibility to the profession and what the occupational therapy team is trying to accomplish. When the occupational therapist works to provide quality evidence and quality data supporting the importance of occupational therapy being involved at all levels of MTSS, the administration will see the credibility and begin to listen to the proposal of the occupational therapy team.

Attitudinal Barriers

While putting forward Knoster's model, the main difficulty when promoting a shift from a traditional caseload approach to a workload approach is ensuring that all team members understand the implementation. Attitudinal barriers are common in educational settings, especially when advocating for change. These can be defined as a mindset or perspective that prevents individuals and organizations from understanding, accepting, or cohesively interacting with others. These barriers often arise from preconceived notions and a lack of knowledge and awareness. Barriers can hinder effective communication, collaboration, and cohesion among educational team members. In most cases, attitudinal barriers in the school setting are due to a lack of knowledge about team member's roles and lack of understanding of how a workload approach is implemented.

Occupational therapists are often only thought of as part of the IEP team in the special education department. As a result, occupational therapy practitioners are often not even considered part of the MTSS team or MTSS planning. This assumes the role of the occupational therapy practitioner and limits the number of students the therapist can serve. The occupational therapist may view themselves only as a direct service provider rather than seeing how essential they can be in meeting the needs of students at the group and population level. Therefore, to enact change in this model, the occupational therapy team must begin to view themselves as part of the whole school team and an important part of the MTSS team for planning and implementing services at all levels.

The school system's MTSS structure lends itself to the occupational therapy team providing services at group and population levels. The occupational therapy practitioner can educate other school personnel, including administrators, on the value of occupational therapy in the MTSS system. However, it takes a systematic approach to facilitate and advocate for lasting change. The occupational therapy practitioner must plan and prepare to begin to help expand the understanding of school administrators on how occupational therapy can be an essential part of general education, not just limited to special education services. Let us take a closer look at how the occupational therapy practitioner may fit into the school team.

Multidisciplinary Teams

Many different disciplines are involved in working with students in the school setting. In addition to teachers and classroom assistants, the school team comprises other professionals, including speech-language pathologists, psychologists, and physical therapists. There are also other teachers beside classroom teachers, such as physical education, music, and art teachers, and support staff, such as cafeteria workers and custodians. All of these individuals play an important role in the day-to-day workings of the school, and each can support the students in unique ways. Learning to work with all school personnel is essential to successfully implementing MTSS programs.

Occupational therapy practitioners work together in school teams that are composed of members of various disciplines. While similar, the multidisciplinary and interdisciplinary teams do have some differences. The multidisciplinary team approaches the client independently based on their expertise. Team members collaborate on the best care for the client but often implement their services separately and independently. Most communication comes via reports and meetings, outside of direct time with the students. Team members work parallel to each other as they focus on their own tasks and areas of expertise. Each team member makes decisions within their own discipline, but the information and outcomes are combined in one comprehensive report.

In an interprofessional team, various disciplines still come together for a common purpose and tend to be more collaborative than a multidisciplinary team. The members work closely together, focusing on their expertise unitedly and holistically. They communicate frequently, support each other's goals within their own expertise, and make decisions as a collective. All education teams are multidisciplinary in nature. Some may function more as an interdisciplinary team (Keshmiri et al., 2021), while others tend to operate more as a multidisciplinary team. However, interdisciplinary teams result in better client outcomes and ease the workload of all team members (Interprofessional Education Collaborative [IPEC], 2023).

There are many ways the occupational therapy practitioner can work closely with other therapy providers to promote an interdisciplinary model for MTSS Tier 1 and Tier 2. Occupational therapists and speech-language pathologists often work collaboratively and closely in many different settings. Since speech-language pathologists are more involved within the school setting than the other therapy disciplines (occupational and physical), they are an excellent starting point for occupational therapy practitioners trying to initiate a collaborative process. Working closely with the speech-language pathologists to incorporate language and social communication goals within the sensory program is a brilliant way to support all students and decrease the burden on teachers and classroom assistants. It also allows occupational therapy practitioners and speech-language pathologists to understand each other's expertise and scope of practice better, and to support each other at all tier levels. Here are some examples of ways to incorporate speech/language goals with sensory supports.

- Supporting spatial concepts while engaging in climbing activities.
- Labeling levels of alertness; describing emotions while engaging in sensory activities.
- Using deep pressure tactile while labeling body parts.
- Describing objects while engaging in visual scanning activities.
- Engaging in movement activities while addressing "wh" questions when students are moving about the school environment (i.e. walking the halls, using a scooter board, etc.).
- Incorporating movement activities into speech sessions.

To truly implement an interprofessional model, speech and occupational therapists must work hard to learn the goals of the other disciplines, and there must be a mutual respect for the expertise of team members. The members of an interprofessional team understand that supporting all goals, with a specific focus on their own discipline, provides the best client outcomes (IPEC, 2023). Further, professionals can support one another and share the workload, which helps prevent burnout.

Working as a multidisciplinary team that is both collaborative and interprofessional requires organizational support. School personnel need time allotted to support interprofessional education through collaboration time and training, and they also need regular access to other professionals. Being intentional about time, space, and purpose in collaboration will help facilitate a true interprofessional practice that extends beyond just collaborative practice. For example, occupational and speech therapists should share office space to support ongoing collaboration. In addition to this, opportunities should be generated to allow people to collaborate, such as scheduled meetings, planning periods, or lunchtimes. Therapists are very busy, so they must be intentional about prioritizing time to collaborate and meet with other professionals. Occupational therapy practitioners can carve out one lunch period a week dedicated to interprofessional planning and be intentional about having lunch with the speech-language pathologist or general education teacher. They can engage in discussions on topics such as sensory and language, sensory and academics, the impact of language on academic achievement, etc. We will now look at this in more detail.

FORMING RELATIONSHIPS WITH SCHOOL PERSONNEL

In the school setting, occupational therapy practitioners' days are frequently hectic, fulfilling requirements for service minutes at a Tier 3 level at different school sites. They typically have high caseloads, high demand for billable hours, and may travel between many schools. As a result, there is limited time for collaboration with staff unless that staff is part of the consultation services minutes, and teachers and school administrators may have limited contact with the occupational therapy practitioners who serve the school. As occupational therapy practitioners frequently travel between buildings and may not be on-site at one school every day, this can make it difficult for teachers and administrators to access the occupational therapist, and even harder for them to form a relationship.

Communication is key in developing relationships with school personnel, and the occupational therapists need to make a special effort. The teacher may see the occupational therapy practitioner as someone who only pulls students from the classroom for IEP minutes rather than seeing them as a collaborator in the educational process. By offering to assist with activities in the classroom and helping teachers and classroom assistants in problem-solving difficult situations or behaviors, the therapist can help change the teacher's perspective. Along with this, the occupational therapist must respect the teacher and their classroom, ensuring that the teacher's opinions and expertise are valued as part of a team. Working with the teacher, the therapist can then identify areas where they have assisted other staff members and be part of the students' progress. The therapist must work to build trust by following through with support and following up with the needs of the teachers and staff. By prioritizing these aspects, the therapist can cultivate positive relationships with all school personnel and contribute to a supportive and productive work environment that supports student needs.

THE ISSUE OF TIME

Lack of time is one of the most frequently reported reasons for therapy staff to not engage in collaborative practice across disciplines. For the occupational therapist, time remains one of the most significant barriers due to caseload size and schedules being established solely around service minutes. However, one solution to time constraints is to work with occupational therapy students.

Having occupational therapy students work directly with children in the classroom allows the licensed therapist to spend more time training and collaborating with teachers and assistants, while still providing supervision. In addition, when staff are adequately trained, the occupational therapy practitioner can oversee many processes and the implementation of sensory strategies rather than being the sole implementor of sensory interventions. Further, any opportunities the occupational therapist has to engage with several school personnel at one time can help maximize time, especially when engaging in training of non-occupational therapy school staff. The use of professional development days allows the occupational therapist to reach many school staff across buildings, thus maximizing the impact of the training time.

COLLECTIVE RESPONSIBILITY

Appreciative inquiry is a method occupational therapy practitioners can use to help build relationships and start conversations with school personnel at all levels (Cooperrider & Whitney, 2005). This method focuses on strengths, possibilities, and what is currently working well rather than what may be problems or areas of need. Using this approach to open the discussion on sensory needs in the district, school, and classroom involves identifying and celebrating sensory preferences and experiences of staff and students. The focus is on sensory experience and preferences that bring joy, comfort, and fulfillment rather than on focusing solely on challenges and deficits in sensory processing. The occupational therapy practitioner would help staff and students understand how sensory experiences positively contribute to a person's well-being and quality of life, with the goal being to help all stakeholders adopt a more holistic and positive perspective on sensory needs in the school setting. By taking time to help other staff understand sensory processing and engage in sensory experiences, the therapist can ensure that staff understand the importance of meeting sensory needs in the classroom and create a sense of collective responsibility.

However, to continue building these relationships and inspire collective teamwork, training is essential.

HOW TO TRAIN SCHOOL PERSONNEL

To effectively implement Tier 1 and Tier 2 interventions, the occupational therapy practitioner must become skilled in training school personnel. One goal of implementing interventions at Tier 1 and Tier 2 is to reduce the burden on the occupational therapy team so they can devote more time to students with higher needs at the Tier 3 level. However, to do this, the occupational therapy team must ensure that school personnel are adequately trained to implement sensory interventions at a population and small group level.

One of the best methods of training is an interactive workshop. This method allows for instruction on the topic to provide background information. Also, it will enable participants to engage in hands-on activities to actively reinforce the content presented. Adding group discussion time during training can allow participants to problem-solve situations and share information. In addition, discussion is an excellent way to check for understanding of the content. Finally, providing case studies or role-playing can facilitate the learning process and ensure that participants understand the information presented.

However, it can be difficult to know how to practically run a training program. Box 7.2 provides an outline of a potential training program for school personnel on sensory integration and processing.

BOX 7.2   INSTRUCTIONAL CONTENT FOR TEACHER/ SCHOOL PERSONNEL TRAINING

A. Background information on sensory integration and processing.
B. How sensory processing impacts learning and behavior.
   a. Regulation of alertness levels.
   b. Body awareness and motor planning.
C. Brief overview of sensory integration theory.
   a. Vestibular.
   b. Proprioceptive.
   c. Tactile.
   d. Auditory.
   e. Visual.
D. Sensory-based interventions.
   a. Examples based on sensory systems.
   b. Examples based on increasing or decreasing alertness level.
   c. How and when to implement.
E. Direct practice of sensory interventions.
F. Case study: Work in small groups to choose from a list of sensory interventions based on students' descriptions and needs.
G. Develop a classroom sensory plan.
   a. Identify sensory tools.
   b. Develop sensory routine/schedule.

Part of effective training is ensuring that school personnel understand the concepts presented and that they can demonstrate understanding. This promotes the fidelity of interventions and builds confidence in their implementation. When teachers and classroom assistants are confident in their ability to implement strategies correctly and effectively, they are more likely to utilize the strategies.

The teach-back method is an evidence-based approach that helps ensure participants understand what they have been taught and reinforces concepts presented in training. In this method, participants are asked to re-teach what they have learned in the session. The concept is to have the participants explain the information in their own words, or "teach-back" to you, the presenter (Agency for Healthcare Research and Quality [AHRQ], 2023). This can be done in pairs, small groups, or large groups.

There are several methods that can be used for teach-back. For example, participants can summarize and share the information from the presentation with the larger group. They can do a pair-in-share, where participants gather in groups of two to three and take turns summarizing the information to "teach" to the other person. The presenter can check that the participants understood the information presented by monitoring the teach-back time. This allows the presenter to clarify or provide information via a different method to help ensure understanding (AHRQ, 2024). During the teach-back, participants should also demonstrate how to implement sensory techniques. This is essential for two reasons. First, it allows the occupational therapist to facilitate the training to ensure the technique is implemented properly. Second, it will enable the participants to experience the sensory techniques in their own bodies and to observe how it impacts their sensory processing and levels of alertness. By experiencing it firsthand, participants can better understand and relate to the sensory strategies and concepts of sensory processing that they will apply to the students they serve. Table 7.1 provides a step-by-step guide to implement the teach-back method within a training session.

When training a large group, breaking the participants into smaller groups based on concepts, such as sensory systems or alerting/calming tools, can be helpful. For example, after explaining each sensory system, you can set up stations for participants to experience different types of movement, such as proprioception, tactile, etc. Having various sensory tools available, and asking teachers to describe how the sensory experience or tool impacts their own arousal level,

Table 7.1 Steps for Teach-Back Method

Steps	Description
Step 1	Describe the concepts Use plain language rather than jargon Define any words/concepts that are not plain language (i.e. vestibular, proprioceptive)
Step 2	Ask questions that promote engagement rather than questions that test the knowledge or retention of knowledge (i.e. "That was a lot of information in a short amount of time. What three things do you think are the most important to remember?")
Step 3	Set up teach-back opportunities • Show-me method demonstration of activities • Large group sharing • Pair and share • Role-play
Step 4	Reteach concepts that need further clarification
Step 5	Provide teach-back opportunities as a second check of understanding

can help support the ideas presented in the training. This provides a way for participants to understand sensory processing related to their body. Allow participants plenty of time to try various techniques to ensure they can perform the technique correctly and that they understand how sensory tools may alert or calm.

Table 7.2 provides a list of some activities that can be used during the training and a chart that allows participants to mark how it makes their body feel. By using these activities during training, the occupational therapist can ensure that the activities are performed correctly and support the concept that each activity may make each participant feel differently.

Table 7.2 Sample Activity List for Staff Sensory Training

Activity	This makes me feel more alert	This makes me feel calmer	This does not seem to impact how I feel
Bouncing on a therapy ball			
Rolling over a therapy ball on your stomach			
Rolling your back over a therapy ball to hang your head backwards			
Using a scooter board on your stomach			
Walking the hallway			
Listening to music			
Using noise-canceling headphones or earplugs			
Listening to white noise			
Using a stress ball			
Using a fidget of choice			
Chewing gum			
Doing a plank or pushups			
Using a weighted blanket or lap pad			
Having someone roll a therapy ball over your body			
Using a sensory bin			
Wearing sunglasses			
Using ankle weights			
Swinging			
Using resistance bands			
Jumping on a trampoline			
Jumping up to touch the door frame 10 times			
Head shakes			
Dancing			
Jumping jacks			
Crab walk, bear walk			

Providing Structured Tiered Interventions with Good Fidelity

As discussed in Chapter 6, good fidelity is essential when implementing interventions at Tier 1 and Tier 2 levels. This is because implementing an intervention without fidelity can cause data to be inaccurate, meaning the observer cannot know whether the intervention was not sound or just poorly implemented. Therefore, it is crucial to ensure that training has good fidelity by following these key components.

1. **Continuous and regular monitoring of performance** ensures that the individuals adhere to the trained protocols and methods. This is often best done through observation or review of written documentation.
2. **Implement a method of feedback** that allows team members to provide input on how they performed the strategies presented.
3. **Refresher training** is an essential component of fidelity checks. Offer periodic refresher training sessions to reinforce the original training and address any gaps or deviations that might have emerged. Create virtual refresher training to provide training opportunities when time is limited.
4. **Establish clearly defined quality assurance measures to assess fidelity** and provide corrective actions when needed. Quality assurance measures may include inspections and observations of the intervention being performed, documentation audits, and gathering feedback from students and those implementing the intervention.
5. **Documentation** is required as part of progress monitoring and allows the occupational therapy practitioner to monitor fidelity without direct observation of the intervention. As part of the progress monitoring, fidelity checks can also be included in the documentation. Examples of quality assurance documentation include how often the intervention was applied and when it was applied. Providing documentation methods with checkboxes for specific key ingredients of the interventions allows those performing the intervention to quickly indicate what methods were utilized in that session. Box 7.3 provides an example of how to include fidelity checks in your progress monitoring documents. This example allows the person providing the deep pressure input to quickly indicate if the input was provided using the key training methods. While not the only form of feedback, this does help the occupational therapist who is monitoring the intervention know if the input was provided as intended. The therapist would also want to know the results of the intervention. Figure 7.1 provides a sample tracking sheet that can be used for this purpose.
6. **Providing leadership support** to help ensure fidelity reinforces the importance of adhering to established practice. Leadership provides accountability to help ensure staff adhere to protocols. Leadership should also be trained

Student(s) Name(s): _____

Date/Time	Staff's Initial's	Activity	Reaction	Comment

Instructions: Note the date and time of the activity. Note what activity was performed. Note the student's reaction as positive or negative, a plus/minus (+/−) sign is sufficient. Any additional comments, write to the side.

Staff Performing Intervention: _____

_____
_____
_____

Figure 7.1 Tracking sheet for sensory input. Image by author.

to answer questions on implementation and help staff solve problems that may arise. They need to help staff know when to seek guidance from the occupational therapist or occupational therapy assistant.

BOX 7.3   FIDELITY CHECK FOR DEEP PRESSURE TACTILE

- The child chose deep pressure tactile (type_____).
- Provided to arms and legs.
- The child appeared/reported positive feelings.
- The child welcomed the input and did not pull away.
- Any redness on the skin disappeared after a few seconds.

By consistently implementing these strategies, occupational therapy practitioners can help maintain the fidelity of interventions over time.

Summary

There is an increase in the need for sensory supports in all areas of the school. By incorporating occupational therapy at each of the MTSS levels, sensory needs can be addressed for all students. However, this requires a shift in thinking from a workload to a caseload model of care. A caseload model provides time and resources for the occupational therapy practitioner to work with students at various MTSS levels while still servicing students who require direct service minutes through an IEP. The shift must come from the occupational therapy practitioner who must garner support from school administration and staff. The occupational therapy team can facilitate organizational change by being systematic about how and when to present information and quality data to school administrators. Further, the multidisciplinary and interprofessional team is key to implementing occupational therapy services at Tier 1 and Tier 2, just as it is at Tier 3. Being intentional about building relationships with other school personnel and carving out designated time to build teams and collaborate on the needs of the school and individual students facilitates a strong MTSS team, with occupational therapy being a key component. Finally, effective training allows the occupational therapy practitioner to share information and interventions with school personnel so they can be effectively integrated into the routines of the school day.

In the final chapter, we will examine the discharge process, explore how occupational therapy looks at each MTSS level, and discuss the future direction of the profession in implementing sensory supports in the school setting.

References

Agency for Healthcare Research and Quality (AHRQ) (2023, February). *Teach-back: Intervention.* https://www.ahrq.gov/patient-safety/reports/engage/interventions/teach-back.html.

Agency for Healthcare Research and Quality (AHRQ) (2024, April). *Use the teach-bask method: Tool 5.* https://www.ahrq.gov/health-literacy/improve/precautions/tool5.html.

American Speech-Language-Hearing Association (2024). *Caseload and workload.* https://www.asha.org/practice-portal/professional-issues/caseload-and-workload/#collapse_1.

Ayres, A. J. (1979). *Sensory Integration and the Child.* Western Psychological Services.

Ben-Sasson, A., Carter, A. S., & Briggs-Gowan, M. J. (2009). Sensory over-responsivity in elementary school: Prevalence and social–emotional correlates. *Journal of Abnormal Child Psychology, 37*, 705–716. https://doi.org/10.1007/s10802-008-9295-8.

Bodison, S. C. & Parham, L. D. (2018). Specific sensory techniques and sensory environmental modifications for children and youth with sensory integration difficulties: A systematic review. *American Journal of Occupational Therapy, 72*(1), 7201190040p1–7201190040p11. https://doi.org/10.5014/ajot.2018.029413.

Cooperrider, D. & Whitney, D. (2011). *Appreciative Inquiry: A Positive Revolution in Change.* Brett-Koehler Publishers.

Cornelius, K. E. & Gustafson, J. A. (2021). Relationships with school administrators: Leveraging knowledge and data to self-advocate. *Teaching Exceptional Children, 53*(3), 206–214. https://doi.org/10.1177/0040059920972438.

Interprofessional Education Collaborative (IPEC) (2023). *IPEC Core Competencies for Interprofessional Collaborative Practice: Version 3*. Interprofessional Education Collaborative.

Jussila, K., Junttila, M., Kielinen, M., Ebeling, H., Joskitt, L., Moilanen, I., & Mattila, M. L. (2020). Sensory abnormality and quantitative autism traits in children with and without autism spectrum disorder in an epidemiological population. *Journal of Autism and Developmental Disorders, 50,* 180–188. https://doi.org/10.1007/s10803-019-04237-0.

Keshmiri, F., Jafari, M., Dehghan, M., Raee-Ezzabadi, A., & Ghelmani, Y. (2021). The effectiveness of interprofessional education on interprofessional collaborative practice and self-efficacy. *Innovations in Education and Teaching International, 58*(4), 408–418. https://doi.org/10.1002/14651858.CD000072.pub3.

Knoster, T. (1991). Presentation in TASH Conference. Washington, D.C.

Kuhn, T. S. (1962). *The Structure of Scientific Revolution.* University of Chicago Press

Lillard, A. S. (2023). Why the time is ripe for an education revolution. *Frontiers in Developmental Psychology,* 1177576. https://doi.org/10.3389/fdpys.2023.1177576.

Rioux, J. E. & Jackson, L. L. (2019). Best practices in determining a workload approach. In G. F. Clarck, J. E. Roius, & B. E. Chandler (eds), *Best Practices for Occupational Therapy in Schools,* 2nd ed, pp.109–118. AOTA Press.

Seruya, F. M. & Garfinkel, M. (2020). Caseload and workload: Current trends in school-based practice across the United States. *American Journal of Occupational Therapy, 74*(5), 7405205090p1–7405205090p8. https://doi.org/10.5014/ajot.2020.039818.

Chapter 8

Changing the Service Model: Facilitating Lasting Change

Introduction

Throughout this book, we have explored how occupational therapy practitioners can contribute to the entire school using a multi-tiered system of supports (MTSS) model. Extending beyond only supporting students in Tier 3, this book has demonstrated how and why occupational therapy should become an important part of Tier 1 and Tier 2 to address the growing sensory needs of the whole student population. For lasting change to occur within the profession – such as reducing stress and burnout in school staff and therapists, improving behavioral and academic performance of students, and making schools run efficiently – occupational therapists should be able to provide sensory supports at all Tier levels. Bringing this all together, we will now examine what occupational therapy looks like when implemented at each Tier level. We will also discuss discharging students from occupational therapy services, and then outline future directions for the field. First, we will begin with one of the most important contributions to the success of an MTSS occupational therapy program: forming a collaborative partnership with teachers.

Forming a Partnership with Teachers

If occupational therapists want to create lasting change by working at all Tier levels, including working in classroom environments at Tier 1, they must learn to work closely, positively, and respectfully with classroom teachers.

Teachers are the leaders of their classrooms, and their role is no small feat. Naturally, we understand that they are responsible for teaching content, offering guidance, and facilitating learning opportunities. However, they also balance many other responsibilities in the management of their classrooms. They ensure classrooms, students, and schedules are organized, that routines are established, and that all students have the resources they need to participate in classroom activities. The teacher is responsible for keeping students on task and engaged in learning, and for maintaining discipline. Teachers provide emotional support

DOI: 10.4324/9781032654768-9

and guidance to students, provide assessment of learning and feedback, and communicate with students and their guardians to facilitate learning and success for all students inside and outside of the classroom.

Occupational therapy practitioners can be a supportive partner to teachers in many ways. They have the knowledge and expertise to provide assistance in supporting positive behaviors, modifying tasks and activities to ensure success for all students, organizing routines to best facilitate learning, and supporting positive mental health. They can also help the classroom teacher as they lead their classroom and students towards success for that academic year. However, for classroom teachers to welcome this assistance, occupational therapists must respect the teacher and their classroom, viewing themselves as a support to the teacher's facilitation and management.

The best way that an occupational therapist can support a teacher, and demonstrate the benefit of their presence in the classroom environment, is by using their understanding of sensory processing and integration to improve the performance and behavior of students in the teacher's class. Most teachers are aware that students have many sensory needs and that providing sensory supports can help students be more attentive and successful in the classroom. When occupational therapy practitioners provide support, especially sensory support, to improve students' attention and on-task behavior, teachers will recognize their value and welcome their contributions. They will be viewed as a facilitator of learning rather than someone who comes to impose their philosophy, telling the teacher how to teach or trying to run their classroom.

The occupational therapy practitioner should be creative when proposing different ways that they can directly and indirectly assist in supporting sensory processing. This requires innovative collaboration between the occupational therapy practitioner and the teacher. Teachers can include sensory supports, as designed by the occupational therapist, in their lessons to embed occupational therapy services within the classroom's daily routine, and the occupational therapy practitioner can arrange their schedule to be in the classroom at times when teachers most need support to address sensory needs.

For example, in lower grades and preschool, learning centers provide an excellent opportunity for the occupational therapy practitioner to come into the classroom and offer support. The occupational therapy practitioner can work with the teacher to set up and facilitate a sensory center to support the sensory needs of all students. On some days, the occupational therapy practitioner can be in the classroom and run the sensory center, providing tailored interventions to the needs of students on their caseload while allowing all students to access sensory strategies. On other days, the occupational therapy practitioner can provide activities to the teacher or assistant to address the classroom's needs (based on information gathered from observation and universal screening). These activities can be set up in an independent sensory center or with a classroom assistant to help facilitate them.

Another way occupational therapy practitioners can support teachers is to have the practitioner build opportunities for sensory input into regular lessons. The occupational therapy practitioner can provide activity suggestions, or if the teacher is open to the idea, help co-teach, providing the sensory component while the classroom teacher conducts the lesson content. The occupational therapy practitioner can assist the teacher in writing lesson plans that include sensory components or assist in the delivery of the lesson at times specified by the teacher. Including sensory-based learning strategies within the lesson plans can provide sensory opportunities for all students, and the occupational therapy practitioner can modify and tailor these activities to students receiving more intensified Tier 2 and Tier 3 services. Table 8.1 includes examples of ways in which occupational therapists can embed sensory input naturally into regular lessons.

Beyond this, there are many simple but transformative ways that the occupational therapist can ensure they are accepted by the teacher. The occupational therapy practitioner must be sensitive to the teacher's needs and make themselves aware of the teacher's goals for and expectations of their students, lessons, and classroom in order to provide the best support possible. As well as this, the occupational therapy practitioner must acknowledge the teacher's hard work managing the classroom and students, and their contributions should try to make the teacher's job easier. Offering assistance in implementing sensory strategies to support classroom management and providing easily accessible tools to support sensory processing is an example of this. Occupational therapy practitioners can make or offer many sensory tools, sensory activity cards, and sensory stations that utilize everyday classroom materials to support sensory needs. If possible, occupational therapists should attend teacher meetings, such as parent-teacher conferences and other staffing meetings. This provides insight into the unique workings of each classroom and the population needs of the classroom. As mentioned in Chapter 7, carving time out of the day to attend meetings can be difficult for occupational therapy practitioners, but even attending part of a meeting for 30 minutes to an hour each week can contribute to making the occupational therapy practitioner feel like part of the school team.

Table 8.1 Sensory-Based Learning Activities

Learning Activity	Example
Writing activities in various media	Salt trays, shaving cream, sandpaper
Math activities with movement	Jumping while counting by 3's
	Skip counting floor mats
Water play	Measuring cups for fractions
Sorting/writing	Place items for sorting in sensory bins and ask students to find an item and match it to a category.
	Place letters in sensory bins and ask students to find a letter and practice letter sounds or writing letters.

Above all, the occupational therapy practitioner must respect the teacher's professional expertise. Teachers have the best interests of the students in mind and tend to know their students' strengths and needs very well. Teachers are also experts in teaching, pedagogy, and classroom management. Encouraging a culture of mutual respect and collaboration helps all staff members feel supported and creates a positive environment to provide respectful feedback and collaboration.

To build a culture of mutual respect, the first step is to lead by example. Even if the occupational therapist disagrees with what and how the teacher implements certain activities in the classroom, they should respect the teacher's expertise. Respect can be demonstrated with small gestures, such as being on time for meetings or scheduled times in the classroom, being polite, and offering compliments. The occupational therapist should look to build a genuine relationship with the teacher, such as getting to know them personally and demonstrating a care for their wellbeing. This can show the teacher that the therapist is a part of their support system. Crucially, especially when there are disagreements, the occupational therapist should ensure they are being an active listener.

Often, differences of opinion may grow from a lack of understanding or lack of knowledge. It is important to remember that teachers and school administrators often have a limited understanding of the scope and training of the occupational therapy practitioner. They may not recognize how many areas the occupational therapy practitioners can address and provide support in. Rather than viewing this as a negative, it should be seen as an opportunity to educate other professionals on the value of occupational therapy.

Finally, celebrate successes together. It is important to acknowledge the contributions of the teacher to the success of the students. If mistakes are made, work to see these as learning opportunities rather than criticizing the approach. Remember, teachers and occupational therapy practitioners are partners, working together to ensure the students' success. When teachers and therapists can come together to implement sensory interventions at all tiers, true, lasting change can occur.

So, how do you begin to build relationships and have effective conversations with teachers? Below are some examples of questions to facilitate discussion surrounding sensory supports and how occupational therapists can help in the classroom environment. This is a sampling of questions to help guide discussion and gain helpful feedback. It should be noted that not all questions should be used due to time constraints, but the list can help the therapist know how to initiate the conversation to gain relevant information in a short amount of time.

- What sensory activities/supports have you implemented?
- Do you feel these sensory activities/supports have helped students?
- What are some barriers to implementing sensory activities/supports that you have experienced?
- Are there sensory activities/supports I have suggested that you still need to implement? Can I provide support to help you do so?

- Are there sensory activities/supports you do not feel are effective? What makes you feel that way?
- Do you have any questions on how suggestions should be implemented?
- How do you feel provided sensory supports are working?
- Are there any suggestions that were provided that you do not use?
- Tell me about the students' progress. Are there any areas of improvement? Areas of concern? Have any areas of progress slowed since the implementation of the sensory activities/suggestions?
- Do you feel excited about the activities/supports I have suggested, or do they feel like a burden?
- What can I do to support you?

Now, before we summarize how to implement sensory supports at all tiers under the MTSS model, let us review some elements that are important to consider at Tier 1: social environmental factors, the physical environment, and funding of sensory equipment.

Social Environmental Factors

Occupational therapy incorporates environmental factors into the physical context, and support and relationships are considered part of the environment. Under the Occupational therapy practice framework: Domain and process–Fourth edition (OTPF-4), support and relationships are defined as "People or animals that provide practical physical or emotional support, nurturing, protection, assistance, and relationships to other persons in the home, workplace, or school or at play or in other aspects of their daily activities" (American Occupational Therapy Association [AOTA], 2020, p. 38). It further designates teachers as persons of authority who serve students when looking at the context of the classroom. Teachers are a part of the environment and bring their own sensory needs and biases to the classroom.

Every person has unique sensory needs, driving different choices during the day. It may be beneficial to help teachers understand their sensory processing and how that drives their choices in setting up their classroom and establishing their classroom routines. For example, a teacher who leans toward the hyperreactive side of processing auditory input may have more rules focused around quiet work time as compared to another teacher who does not have any hyperreactivity to auditory input. Other teachers may not have auditory sensitivities and may structure their classroom routines to have more time allotted in the day for group work and group discussions. Often teachers are not aware of how their sensory preferences impact the set-up of their classrooms and how they like to manage their class.

It may be beneficial to recommend a teacher carry out a sensory assessment on themselves to see how this impacts their choices in the classroom. If a teacher's sensory preferences differ significantly from students in the classroom, the teacher can be mindful of these differences to set up spaces with other types of sensory input. Occupational therapists may want to incorporate sensory screening or sensory assessment for teachers during professional development training or when initially assessing the classroom environment to provide Tier 1 support. This information can help the teacher be more aware of sensory processing and how their sensory choices affect the setup and routines of the classroom. It can also help teachers understand sensory processing, and how their sensory preferences drive their choices, just they drive the student's choices.

Physical Environment of the Classroom and Sharing Sensory Resources

As outlined, teachers are responsible for the physical set-up of the classroom, and the occupational therapist must respect the structure and boundaries of the learning environment. However, they can also provide simple suggestions to help teachers design a sensory inclusive classroom that meets the needs of their students. The occupational therapy team can share resources with classroom teachers and design methods for teachers to share sensory tools. This can be done through a lending library.

A lending library format allows teachers to "check out" larger pieces of sensory equipment for a specified time. This serves two purposes. First, teachers can meet the short-term sensory needs of students or the classroom and then return the equipment to the library. Since sensory needs vary and change frequently, and the nervous system adapts over time, this can be a very helpful model. Sometimes repetitive sensory input or the same environmental modification provided over and over causes the nervous system to adapt to that input, making it no longer effective. Instead, teachers can change sensory tools regularly to allow for novelty in the sensory input to help prevent neurological adaptation to the point that the input is no longer effective. The lending library is also a cost-effective alternative to every classroom needing to purchase its own sensory equipment as sharing resources promotes collaboration and saves money.

BOX 8.1   SENSORY LENDING LIBRARIES

Items to consider for a sensory lending library:

- rocking chairs
- therapy balls
- t-stools
- vestibular discs
- cube chairs

- fidgets
- various swatches of fabric
- swings
- mini trampoline
- balance board
- weighted blankets
- weighted lap pads
- ankle weights
- scooter boards
- light covers
- lamps
- lava and bubble lamps
- noise machines
- noise-dampening items (i.e. fabric squares, curtains, carpet squares or rugs, etc.).

The occupational therapy team needs to oversee the resources to ensure the best tools are available and used in accordance with the needs of the students. Remember, providing general sensory equipment is not best practice and not effective in managing sensory needs. Instead, the occupational therapist needs to assess the needs of the client (population, group, or individual) to provide the best sensory tools for the needs of the students. Further, the occupational therapy team should work to ensure organization of the equipment. They may consider consulting with the school librarian to establish a check out procedure. Equipment should also be checked on a regular basis as part of the checking in/out process to ensure the equipment is in good working order and is safe and clean for use.

As part of the lending library, the occupational therapy team can provide equipment suggestions per classroom. After universal screenings, the occupational therapist will have an idea of what type of sensory input is needed for each classroom, providing a list to each teacher so they understand what best fits the needs of their class. Box 8.2 provides an example of an equipment list that was developed as a result of an occupational therapist's participation in the universal screening process.

BOX 8.2   EXAMPLE OF LENDING LIBRARY SUGGESTIONS FOR MR. ROBERT'S SECOND GRADE CLASSROOM

Suggested equipment:

- vestibular discs
- balance boards

- rocking chairs
- weighted items.

Guidelines: Students need some additional movement during seated activities. Providing vestibular discs, balance boards, and rocking chairs can allow students the opportunity to increase movement without over-stimulating their nervous systems. Having weighted items available can help students attend to instructional time and calm after returning from recess.

Funding for Sensory Tools

Funding can be difficult in the school setting where budgets are often limited; sensory tools may not be high on the list of priorities when budgets are tight. As noted in the previous section, sensory tools can be expensive and it is in the occupational therapist's interest to find creative ways to obtain and share these resources.

Here are some ideas to help with funding sensory materials for classrooms.

- **Parent-teacher organization (PTO)**: The PTO supports classroom teachers and helps provide funds for many supplies not covered by school budgets. This can be an excellent way to provide funding for sensory tools.
- **University occupational therapy programs**: University occupational therapy programs often have student projects and assignments where students need to make therapy equipment. Contact your local university to see if there is a way to collaborate with the students; the students could either make sensory equipment or fundraise to help buy sensory equipment.
- **Career tech classes**: Career Tech classes can help make sensory tools such as T-stools, scooter boards, balance boards, etc. as part of their curriculum.
- **Donations/school supply lists**: Talk with parents and teachers about donating small sensory items, such as items for sensory bins (e.g., rice, beans, etc.), fidgets, and weighted items. Parents may often be able to provide small items as part of their school supply list. There may also be parents who are experts in sewing who would be willing to make sensory items for the classroom.
- **Budget**: Ask school administrators for a small budget for sensory tools. As sensory supports are implemented, the occupational therapist can use the data gathered through progress monitoring to show the importance of sensory tools. This information can be presented to administrators to ask for a budget to purchase more equipment and supplies.

Implementation of Sensory Supports under MTSS

The implementation of sensory supports under each MTSS tier considers several factors, including the environment, the attitudes and acceptance of those within the environment, and training for those implementing the sensory support. Now, we will review how to implement sensory supports in each of the Tier levels by examining the environment, attitudes, and training that should be addressed when implementing a comprehensive sensory support program in the school setting.

Tier 1: Population

Environmental

- Changes in lighting, including natural lights, lamps, light covers, dimmable lights.
- Noise dampening items (pillows, curtains, sound reduction panels, etc.).
- Alternative seating options for students to choose from (balls, rocking chairs, stools, standing, etc.).
- Embedding movement and heavy work into routines throughout the day.
- Providing visual supports that offer sensory suggestions for students to choose from and engage in as needed throughout the day.

Attitudinal

- Students have different preferences and needs for learning. To create the ideal learning environment, some prefer more stimulation, and others prefer less. By creating different spaces and options, students can choose what is best for their learning style.
- Providing sensory tools is not a distraction to learning but a facilitator. If students are not using the sensory tools to facilitate learning, it is a good indication that they do not need the tools.
- Implementing cognitive-based self-regulation programs, such as Zones of Regulation or The Alert Program, to encourage students to become independent in meeting their sensory needs to promote optimal learning.

Training

- Providing an introduction to sensory processing and how sensory processing impacts alertness levels on professional development days.
- Providing written guidelines and options for sensory tools and sensory environmental supports for teachers to implement on a school or classroom-wide level.

- Carrying out fidelity checks (observations) throughout the year through progress monitoring.
- Being a support to all school personnel, answering questions and providing additional training and modeling as needed.

Example of Tier 1

Ms. Finch was teaching second grade. She wanted to attempt to implement sensory supports within her classroom to help meet the needs of all students and provide sensory input to the students in her classroom, including those who received special education and those who did not.

First, Ms. Finch consulted with the school occupational therapist. The occupational therapist worked with Ms. Finch before the school year began and provided basic training on how sensory processing impacts levels of alertness and attention. The occupational therapist also helped assess the current classroom environment and suggested creating spaces with increased sensory stimulation and areas with decreased sensory stimulation. For areas with less stimulation, Ms. Finch put fabric boards (homemade sound reduction panels) on the walls with plain colored fabrics to soak up the sounds and reduce the amount of visual stimulation. She also put light covers over the overhead lights. She created a separate space with bookshelves to separate the area from the rest of the classroom. In this space, she had a basket of weighted items and a basket of fidgets for students to use as needed. Packages of disposable earplugs and noise-canceling headphones were also made available in this space. She provided beanbag chairs and lap desks as an alternative to regular school desks. Ms. Finch also created a more stimulating space in a separate area of the classroom. This space had bright colors and bulletin boards on the walls. She provided options for seating, including stability balls, vestibular discs, and standing desks.

After the school year began, the occupational therapist performed three classroom observations at different times during the day. She also provided sensory questionnaires to the students and Ms. Finch to determine the sensory needs of the class. With that information, the occupational therapist helped Ms. Finch develop a classroom routine that provided movement at various intervals and heavy work at other times to match the classroom tasks and sensory processing needs throughout the day. The occupational therapist built in time to check on the classroom and engage in unstructured interviews with Ms. Finch every month to monitor progress and help identify if students needed additional support.

Let us pause for a moment and look at the role of occupational therapy in social and emotional learning supports as a Tier 1 intervention.

Occupational Therapy Services as Social and Emotional Learning Supports

Social and emotional learning (SEL) is an educational framework that promotes positive mental health, positive behavior, and social participation for students. It is part of the standard public-school curriculum embedded in general education. Some key components of SEL curriculums include self-awareness, self-management, social awareness, relationship skills, and responsible decision-making (Collaborative for Academic, Social, and Emotional Learning [CASEL], 2024). The goals of an SEL program include the following.

- Understand, recognize, and manage emotions.
- Learn what constitutes a positive relationship, how to develop communication skills, and how to develop and maintain positive relationships.
- Understand social cues, respect diversity, and show respect and empathy for others.
- Productively manage conflicts, manage stress and anxiety, and develop resilience.

Occupational therapy has its foundation in mental health and views mental health promotion as part of the core construct of occupational therapy. Many students with sensory sensitivities also have poor psychological health and increased anxiety (Bang et al., 2024; Takahashi et al., 2020). Occupational therapy practitioners can support school-wide mental health through the MTSS model using sensory supports as part of the larger SEL curriculum. The occupational therapy team can promote sensory strategies and understanding of sensory processing to provide positive behavioral support and emotional management. They can help school systems design and promote environments that allow for sensory regulation and help teachers and other professionals learn relaxation techniques that can be incorporated into the school day (AOTA, 2024).

Embedding sensory training, sensory techniques, and relaxation and mindfulness techniques into the SEL curriculum is an excellent way for occupational therapy to intervene at the Tier 1 level to support social and emotional learning. Here are some examples of activities for Tier 1 supports for SEL that incorporate sensory techniques, and that occupational therapists can oversee the training and implementation of.

- Incorporating regulation curriculums into the school curriculum (i.e. Zones of Regulation (Kuypers, 2011); Teen Anxiety Program (Piller & Rooney, 2024)).
- Planning school-wide relaxation times with meditation, calming music, and deep-pressure tactile once a day for 15–20 minutes. This promotes relaxation and mindfulness, while meeting sensory needs.
- Creating calming spaces outside the classroom with sensory tools for students to retreat to if they need a break, become anxious, or feel overwhelmed.

- Incorporating curriculums to help students understand their body signals through interoception (Mahler, 2019).
- Assisting with trauma-informed care approaches, specifically the sensory regulation aspect of programs such as Trust Based Relational Intervention® (TBRI) (Purvis et al., 2013).
- Promoting opportunities for movement, breathing, and mindfulness as part of the regular school routine and teaching students how to incorporate these into their regular daily routines.
- Working with physical education teachers to develop movement programs that promote active movement and mindfulness during the school day and before and after school. Activities such as nature walks, sensory walks, and yoga are opportunities to promote mindfulness with movement and are also regulating.
- Helping students understand their triggers and gain strategies for calming input in a variety of situations and school environments.

Tier 2: Group

Environmental

- Small areas of the classroom or school that are designed for specific sensory needs, such as a space for those who are hyporeactive and those who are hyperreactive.
  - Hyporeactive space: Movement equipment such as stability balls, trampolines, and swings; posted exercises with weight-bearing activities for students to engage in; tactile tools such as sensory bins, swatches of fabric, and crash pads; speakers for music; visual stimulation such as bubble lights, strobe lights, party lights.
  - Hyperreactive space: Rocking chairs, scooter boards, crash pads, weighted items, headphones, low-level lighting.

Specified movement and heavy work routines to be designed around the time of day when students need extra input.

- Student toolboxes for cognitive-based regulation programs with options for students to choose from to meet their needs. Activities that can be done as a group can also promote social participation.

Attitudinal

- Although group sensory sessions may reduce students' instructional time in the classroom, their instructional time will be more effective if they are in a regulated state.

- Providing learning activities while students are engaging in sensory activities to support the main classroom instructional time content.
- Sensory groups can be performed during independent work time, and shortened assignments can be offered so students do not miss instructional or work time.
- Using students in upper grades to help facilitate groups for students in lower grades can allow the teacher or classroom assistant more time to focus on academics rather than facilitating sensory groups.

Training

- Train teachers on designing sensory group activities based on the students' needs. The occupational therapy practitioner can create a list of five or six sensory groups and train the teacher or teacher assistant on how they implement each group. They can rotate these activities each day.
- Train teachers on how to place students in groups based on student sensory processing needs.
- Offer a variety of options for sensory input that can be used in the classroom and group settings.
- Train teachers to incorporate students with Tier 3 needs into the Tier 2 groups. For example, a student receiving support under Tier 3 with goals to address social participation and motor planning could lead a gross motor sensory group for students serviced under Tier 2.

Example of Tier 2

The fourth grade teachers collectively identified a group of students with sensory needs that impacted their ability to participate fully in classroom activities. There were two to three students from each class who were identified during the universal screening process, which received assistance from the occupational therapist. The fourth grade teachers worked with the occupational therapist to design two sensory spaces that all fourth grade classrooms could use. One space had sensory tools that were more stimulating for students who tended to be more hyporeactive to sensory input. The other space was a calming, quiet space for students who may experience overstimulation.

The occupational therapist performed classroom observations to assess the classroom routines and when students may need additional sensory supports. The therapist also provided a sensory questionnaire to the students so they could indicate their sensory preferences and needs during the school day. With this information, the occupational therapist designed specific sensory activities that would meet the needs of Tier 2 students. The occupational therapist created a book of activities for these students to choose from when they needed sensory input and worked with the classroom teacher to develop a routine for the whole class regarding the best time for sensory breaks based on the classroom needs. Students identified as needing Tier 2 interventions used the specialized sensory areas that the fourth grade classrooms had created. Within these areas, the students had access to choices for sensory activities specifically designed for their needs. The occupational therapist utilized the book of sensory activities to provide sensory choices, and the students used the equipment in the sensory spaces, choosing activities from their books and reporting how these made their bodies feel.

The tracking in their sensory books allowed the occupational therapist to monitor their progress and adjust their sensory activities as needed. By providing more targeted sensory input in a small group setting simultaneously with the classroom sensory breaks, the students in Tier 2 could have their sensory needs met.

Tier 3: Individual

At Tier 3 (individual) in the school setting, students receive services under an individualized education program (IEP). This allows the occupational therapist to provide direct and indirect services and supports tailored to the individual student's unique needs. The occupational therapist should work with the other IEP team members to embed sensory supports throughout the student's school day. Since Tier 3 interventions are also supported by Tier 1 and Tier 2, the opportunity to provide sensory supports should already be in the classroom and small group settings. In this case, the occupational therapist can provide specified supports for the students receiving Tier 3 interventions.

However, if effective interventions are in place at the Tier 1 and Tier 2 level, students may not need as much direct one-on-one time to address sensory needs. Instead, occupational therapy practitioners can focus more on students with higher needs or other needs outside of sensory processing. Additionally, the time devoted to one-on-one interventions can be focused on the higher needs of the student that cannot be met in a group or population setting. The occupational therapist can also work with Tier 1 and Tier 2 interventions to ensure options for students receiving Tier 3 interventions are available and that staff are trained on how to encourage these more individualized interventions for the students with higher levels of needs.

For example, if the class engages in a movement break, the occupational therapist can instruct the teacher or classroom aide to encourage a particular student to spend this time in the sensory room doing some swinging to get more intensified vestibular input. This embeds the intervention within the regular classroom routine and allows the student to get their higher sensory needs met in a more specific manner without taking away from instructional time, since it is at the same time the other students are also taking a movement break.

If interventions are successful at different tier levels, and students are shown to improve academically and behaviorally, students can start to be discharged from occupational therapy services. We will now see how this can take place according to best practice.

Discharge from Occupational Therapy Services

When students receive services under Tier 3, interventions often resemble occupational therapy interventions in medical settings, with recurring treatment sessions that work towards goal achievement and eventually discharge from occupational therapy services. Yet, when working with students, occupational therapy services may be in place for years. Since the Individuals with Disabilities Education Act (IDEA) only requires a re-evaluation every three years, often supports are in place until the re-evaluation, although frequency and service minutes may change with each new annual IEP. Parents and teachers may see their child make great improvements and become successful in school with the IEP supports, including occupational therapy, in place. This is often contrary to how their child was performing prior to the initiation of services under the IEP. If their child is doing well with the supports, parents may be reluctant to discontinue those services even though the child is doing well and has met their goals. Therefore, one benefit of having an occupational therapist as a member of the MTSS team is that occupational therapy services do not end when a child is discharged from Tier 3 services. Instead, the services continue, just in a different Tier and with less intensity.

When supports are in place under a Tier 1 and Tier 2 model, discharge and transition from Tier 3 occupational therapy services is easy. Students can be discharged from Tier 3 into Tier 2 to ensure they still receive additional support, but not in an intensified or individualized manner. This can help ease the transition from intensified support and provide a bridge so that students are not left without support entirely. Instead, there is a gradual reduction in the support provided as the student moves towards independence. This can help ensure student success without direct services as the occupational therapist can continue monitoring the student and provide support. Additionally, this can ease the minds of parents who may be reluctant to pull back on support when their child is finally successful in the school setting.

When a child is discharged from Tier 3 occupational therapy services, the occupational therapist can develop a plan for Tier 2 interventions as part of the discharge planning process. This would need to include a profile of their sensory processing, what sensory tools are effective, and when sensory supports should be implemented. The occupational therapist can determine which sensory group already established at the Tier 2 level would be best for this student and develop a schedule for the student to join that group time. The occupational therapist will continue to support the Tier 2 group and monitor data collected in the progress monitoring process. If changes in support are needed, the occupational therapist will know immediately and be able to implement support to ensure the student's continued success. However, for this to happen effectively, documentation must have been ongoing throughout the student's occupational therapy support.

We will now look at the future directions of the field to benefit the whole student population, therapists, and school personnel.

Future Directions for Occupational Therapy

For over 100 years, occupational therapy practitioners have been servicing clients with a variety of needs to support participation and improved function. Their unique skillset allows them to see the person in a holistic manner with a specialized understanding of how the mind and body work together and influence one another. They are the only profession that has specified training in the neurological processes of sensory integration, how sensory processing influences learning and behavior, and direct training on sensory integration therapy, including sensory techniques and Ayres Sensory Integration® (Dean et al., 2019).

Many students have unmet sensory needs that influence their participation in the classroom. However, throughout this book, we have seen that occupational therapy services can be implemented according to many different methods and do not only have to be implemented in a one-on-one model. Occupational therapy is well equipped as a profession to service students at all three levels of the MTSS model: population, group, and individual. In fact, many students' sensory needs are better serviced at a population or group level rather than an individual level. The only way we can help as many students as possible while lessening the pressure on schools and staff is by implementing sensory support in lower tiers, reducing the amount of individualized support needed and moving away from a caseload model. By establishing sensory supports in the daily routine of students and teachers, this promotes the use of sensory supports in other areas of life and facilitates the integration of sensory strategies into the daily routines of the students, both in school and out of school.

Occupational therapists should take the lead on implementing sensory supports into the MTSS model. This can be done through advocacy, research, and practice. With advocacy, occupational therapy practitioners can work with MTSS administrators to define the role and scope of practice for occupational therapy to support learning and positive behavioral support at each Tier level. In research, occupational therapists should lead the way in establishing procedures to examine the effectiveness of sensory environmental modifications, sensory-based interventions, and training for teachers on providing sensory supports in order to establish guidelines and protocols for how to best implement sensory supports in the school setting under each MTSS level. As occupational therapists develop progress monitoring methods for sensory supports, this data can be used to help contribute to a more formal research process. Collaboration with university occupational therapy programs can allow the data already collected to be used in research projects to retrospectively or prospectively examine implementation procedures and effectiveness.

Finally, the practice of occupational therapy needs to shift thinking from an individualized service model to addressing the needs of the entire school population. Implementing school-wide sensory supports affords all students the opportunity to have their sensory needs met for optimal learning and engagement. Even when occupational therapy is not yet involved in the MTSS process, collaboration with classroom teachers of students receiving Tier 3 services can be a great starting point for implementing classroom-wide interventions. By addressing advocacy, research, and practice, occupational therapy can make a lasting change in how sensory supports are implemented in the school setting and support all students in their effort to learn and thrive in the school environment.

Summary

Changes in thinking and philosophy can be difficult for all parties involved. There are many barriers that occupational therapy practitioners and schools face in the switch to implementing occupational therapy services at MTSS Tier 1 and Tier 2 rather than just at Tier 3. It can be challenging to shift from a more medical model of one-on-one treatment to providing skilled interventions in a population model. However, given the sensory needs of so many students today, implementing tailored sensory interventions within the day-to-day routines of the school day has the potential to improve academic performance, school climate, and teacher satisfaction.

Throughout this book we have taken a look at how occupational therapy can service all students. The MTSS model provides the framework for occupational therapy to provide the needed sensory interventions and environmental supports for all students, not just those with more significant individualized needs. With proper support, training, and collaboration, occupational therapy can address the sensory needs of all students. As a result, occupational therapy practitioners will have more time to devote to individuals with more significant needs, reducing burnout and promoting student success.

Now is the time to promote occupational therapy as a standard in MTSS to support sensory needs and promote learning and positive behavior.

References

American Occupational Therapy Association (AOTA) (2020). Occupational therapy practice framework: Domain and process–Fourth edition. *American Journal of Occupational Therapy*, *74*(S2), 1–85. https://doi.org/10.5014/ajot.2020.74S2001.

American Occupational Therapy Association (AOTA) (2024). *School mental health toolkit.* https://www.aota.org/practice/clinical-topics/school-mental-health-toolkit.

Ayres, A. J. (1979). *Sensory Integration and the Child.* Western Psychological Services.

Bang, P., Andemichael, D. K., Pieslinger, J. F., & Igelström, K. (2024). Sensory symptoms associated with autistic traits and anxiety levels in children aged 6–11 years. *Journal of Neurodevelopmental Disorders, 16*(1), 45. https://doi.org.10.1186/s11689-024-09562-9.

Collaborative for Academic, Social, and Emotional Learning (CASEL) (2024). *What is the CASEL framework?* https://casel.org/fundamentals-of-sel/what-is-the-casel-framework/.

Dean, E. E., Little, L. M., Wallisch, A., & Dunn, W. (2019). Sensory processing in everyday life. In B. A. Boyt Schell & G. Gillen (eds), *Willard and Spackman's Occupational Therapy*, 4th ed., pp. 942–964. Wolters Kluwer.

Kuypers, L. (2011). *The Zones of Regulation.* Social Thinking Publishing.

Mahler, K. (2019). *The Interoception Curriculum: A Step-by-Step Guide to Developing Mindful Self-Regulation.* (n.p)

Purvis, K. B., Cross, D. R., Dansereau, D. F., & Parris, S. R. (2013). Trust-based relational intervention® (TBRI): A systematic approach to complex developmental trauma. *Child & Youth Services, 34*(4), 1–28. https://doi.org/10.1080/0145935X.2013.859906.

Piller, A. & Rooney, D. A. (2024). *Teen Anxiety Program.* (n.p.)

Takahashi, T., Kawashima, I., Nitta, Y., & Kumano, H. (2020). Dispositional mindfulness mediates the relationship between sensory-processing sensitivity and trait anxiety, well-being, and psychosomatic symptoms. *Psychological Reports, 123*(4), 1083–1098. https://doi.org/10.1177/0033294119841848.

Index

Note: Locators in *italic* indicate figures, in **bold** tables, and in ***bold-italic*** boxes.

504 Plan 16, **16**, 74–75, 182

action and expression as UDL component 19, 20
Alert Program® for Self- Regulation 47, 146, 147, 212
alertness levels 36, 117–120, **119–120**, 146–147, 149, *197*
American Occupational Therapy Association (AOTA) 83, 187
arousal levels 32, 36, **37**, 120, **120–121**, 136, 149, 154
assessments in occupational therapy 78–112, 157–160; accuracy criteria 80–81; Ayre Sensory Integration® (ASI) **42**; case study (Sarah) *81*, 82–83; child's perspective 106–107, *107–108*; classroom routines and physical/social features 21–22; criterion-referenced assessments **89**, 157, 158; defining, functions 79–80; direct 105–106; evaluation vs assessment 78–80; IEP 74; initial, pre-intervention 83–84; methods 63, 80, 82–83; needs 94–95; norm-referenced 157–158; observations (*see under own heading*); outcomes (proximal, distal) 91; performance-based 87, **88**; psychometric properties 158–159; questionnaires 104, **104**; sensory needs 63; sensory reactivity/ modulation 85–86, **86**; standardized, non-standardized 80, 83, **86**, 87, 104, 112, 157–158; steps, forms 94; task–activity transition 88–90, **89**; top-down,

bottom-up 85; variety need 80–81, 82; *see also* evaluation sensory processing
assessments measures, criteria 80–81, 159–160; concurrent validity 160; construct validity 160; content validity 160; fidelity 168–169; predictive validity 160; reliability 81, 91, 158, 159; validity 159–160
auditory sensory system, environment, stimulation/activities 33, 38, **44**, 45–46, **91**, **131**, 142
autism, case example *176*
Ayres Sensory Integration® (ASI): components 41, **42**; effectivity, fidelity assessment 43, 122; Evaluation in Ayres Sensory Integration® (EASI) 82, **86**, **88**; MTSS tiers applicability 124; purpose, goals principles 21, 41, 124; sensory integration and processing theory (A. Jean Ayres) 30–33, 41–43, 47, 61; sensory ladders 148; teacher-training dependence 47

baseline data 13, 65, 66, 157, 171–172
body awareness 32, 34, 120, 137, 144, 215
Bruininks-Oseretsky Test of Motor Proficiency–Third Edition (BOT-3) **88**

case studies: autism (Annabelle) *176*; evaluation process (Sarah) *81*, 82–83; evaluation synthesis (Meredith) *110–111*; inclusive education support, classroom settings *25–26*; sensory

processing differences, impact
(Anthony) *39–41*
Center on Multi-Tiered Systems of
Support 167, 168
central nervous system (CNS) 34, 41
Classroom Sensory Environment
Assessment (C-SEA) **104**
client-centered care model and evaluation
164–165
clinical utility 157, 160
*Clinician's Guide for Implementing
Ayres Sensory Integration®: Promoting
Participation for Children with Autism*
(Schaaf and Mailloux) 122
coaching, teacher; *see* training school
personnel
cognitive energy, capacity 38–39, *40*, 110
cognitive tasks 117–118
cognitive testing 101, 104
cognitive-based regulation programs 134,
145–150; Alert Program 146, 147, 212;
implementation in intervention plans
150, **151**, 152–153, **153**, 212; Sensory
Ladders 148–149, *150*; Zones of
Regulation 146–148, *148*, **176**, 212
concurrent validity, assessment
measures 160
consistency evaluation, assessment,
data: internal, outcome measures 159;
intervention fidelity 159, 169–170,
201; progress monitoring 65, 127;
testing 159
construct validity, assessment
measures 160
consultation services 175
content validity, assessment measures 160
criterion-referenced assessments **89**,
157, 158

data (collection, quality, use): baseline
data 13, 65, 66, 157, 171–172; data
sheets, plots *23*, 65, 168 *169*, *171*,
201; decision making (interventions,
treatment) 52, 60, 65–67, 74, 171–172,
172–174; frequency, gathering
timelines 61, 65, 171–172; progress
monitoring 52, 65–67, 127, 167–168,
169, 170–171; quality 170–171; sense
making process 67–70, 74; synthesis
of evaluation data 108–109, **109**;
time/resource advocacy 186; training,

collection and handling *26*; types 67,
68; universal screening 54, 163–164
data-driven decision-making (DDDM) 70,
122, 123
deficit intervention model 165
discharge 174–175, 218–219
distal outcomes 85, 90–93, **91**, *92*, 106,
108, 109, **123**, 168
distance sensory systems 33
drawing activities, occupational
profiling *96*
Dunn, Winnie 125

early intervening services 6, 11–12,
14, 126
Ecology of Human Performance (EHP)
125–126
Education for All Handicapped Children
Act (EHA, 1975) (Public Law
94–142), 6–7
engagement, student/client motivation, as
UDL component 18, 19–20, 21, 47, 72,
85, 118; *see also* stimulation
environment; *see* sensory environment
evaluation sensory processing 78–112;
case studies (Meredith) *110–111* /
(Sarah) *81*, 82–83; child's perspective
inclusion 106–108, *107–108*;
evaluation synthesis 78, *79*, 108–110;
evaluation vs assessment 79–80;
IDEA evaluation process and criteria
80–81; methods 82–83; occupational
performance analysis 78, 86, 97–106,
108–109 (*see also under own heading*);
occupational profiles 78–79, 93–95,
95–96, **95**, 97; occupational therapist's
role 82–83, 111; outcomes and goal
setting 85–87, 90–93, 108–109,
111–112 (*see also* outcomes); as
pre-intervention necessity 83–84;
purpose 78
Every Student Succeeds Act (ESSA,
2015) 3, 13–14, 70; *see also* multi-
tiered system of supports (MTSS)
expression and action as UDL component
19, 20

Family Educational Rights and Privacy
Act (FERPA, 1974) 15–16
fidelity, interventions 41–43, **42**, 124,
168–170, 172–173, 197, 200–201, 213

fidgets 140, *141*
fight, flight, or freeze response 31, 33, 35
floor and ceiling effects 158, 160
focus groups 94, 101
FRAME (framework for reporting
    adaptations and modifications to
    evidence-based interventions) 69
free and appropriate education
    (FAPE) 7–8
free play 140, 142, 144–145, 179
frequency counts 65, 161, 163–164,
    168, *169*
future directions 219–220

games, occupational profiling 61, 94, 95,
    95–96, 97
goal setting, MTTS 127–129, *128*;
    example *128*; Tier 1 127, 128–129; Tier
    2 127, 128, 129, 136; SMART goal
    111; *see also* intervention design
Goal-Oriented Assessment of Life Skills
    (GOAL) 82, **88**, 162
gustatory sensory system 34, **37**

headphones *132–133*
Health Insurance and Portability and
    Accountability Act (HIPAA, 1996)
    15–16
How Does Your Engine Run? (Williams
    and Schellenberg) 146
Human Bingo, game *95–96*
hyperreactivity 35, 39, 90, 116, 119–120,
    130, 132, 151–152, 208, 215
hyporeactivity 35, 36, 38–39, 90, 116,
    130, 132, 215

inclusive education 18–19, 21–22;
    acceptance, attitudinal shifts towards
    23–25, *25–26*; barriers 18–19; case
    study *25–26*; concept, definition 18;
    vs least restrictive environment (LRE)
    18; occupational therapist's roles 18,
    21–22, 23–25; setting development
    18–19
independent educational evaluation (IEE)
    8, 10
Individualized Education Plan (IEP)
    8–11; vs 504 Plan **16**, 74, 182; case
    example (Anabelle) *176*; components
    10, **10**, 11; IEP teams 10, 11; legal
    foundation (IDEA, 1990/2004) 8;

MTSS (Tier 3) 51, 62–63, *62*, 74, 111,
    175, 217; occupational therapist's role
    17, 51, 180, 180–181, 185; service
    time allotment 180–181, 183; updates,
    discharge 218
Individualized Family Service Plan
    (IFSP) 12
Individuals with Disabilities Education
    Act (IDEA, 1990/2004) 6–12; aim,
    impact 6; early intervening services
    11–12; EHA as precursor (1975)
    6–7; eligibility 8, **9**; individualized
    education programs (IEPs) 11 (*see also
    under own heading*); Individualized
    Family Service Plans (IFSPs) 12; least
    restrictive environment (LRE) 6, 11,
    18, 126; multi-tiered system of supports
    (MTSS) (*see under own heading*);
    related service, occupational therapy as
    6–7, 11–12; Response to Intervention
    (RTI) 13, 14, 50, 175, **188–189**
Individuals with Disabilities Education
    Act (IDEA, 1990/2004), parts/
    sections 7–12; 2004 reauthorization
    and expansion 12; Part A (free and
    appropriate education, FAPE access
    rights) 7–8, **9**; Part B (implementation,
    IEPs, LRE) 8, 10–11, **10** (*see also
    individualized education programs
    (IEPs)*); Part C (early intervention
    services) 11–12; transitional services
    11; whole school approach 8
internal consistency 159
interoception 34, **37**
interprofessional teams and perspectives
    193–194
interrater reliability 159
intervention design 115–154; auditory
    131, 132, *132–133*, 141; cognitive-
    based regulation programs 134,
    145–150 (*see also under own heading*);
    free play, recess 140, 142, 144–145,
    179; goal setting 127–129; olfactory
    131; proprioceptive **131**, 137–139;
    sample sensory program *143*; sensory
    environment modification 129–134
    (*see also* sensory environment,
    designing and modifications); sensory
    processing and alertness levels 36,
    117–120, **120–121**, 146–147, 149;
    sensory processing patterns 115–117;

student-centered approach 164–165; tactile **131**, 133–134, *134*, *135*, 139–140, *141*; theoretical approaches, choosing 121–126; vestibular **131**, 136–137; visual 130–132, **131**, 142

intervention design, MTSS/Tier 1: development considerations 70–71, 117; examples 59, 151; intervention target, goal setting 14, **57**, 58–59, 127, 128–129; sensory environment interventions, designing and modifications 51, 59–60, 63, 68, 70, 97, 122, 134–136, 150–151, *152*

intervention design, MTSS/Tier 2: development considerations 72–73, **73**; examples 153, **153**; intervention target, goal setting 127, 128, 129, 136; sensory environment interventions, designing and modifications 60, 97, 117, 122, 134–136, 151–153, **153**

intervention design, MTSS/Tier 3: intervention target, goal setting 15, **57**, 62, 74–75; sensory environment interventions, designing and modifications 73, 117

intervention outcome evaluation 156–177; consultation services 175; criterion-referenced assessments **89**, 157, 158; norm-referenced assessments 157–158; outcome measure definition steps 156–157, 177; outcome types and reporting 160–164 (*see also* outcomes); positive behavior interventions and support (PBI&S) plan 166–167, 177; progress monitoring (*see under own heading*); psychometric properties 112, 157, 158–160, 163, 177; reliability types, measures 159; student-centered approach 20–21, 164–166

interviews 87, 94–95, 97, 100–102, 103, *103*, 106

Knoster Model for Managing Complex Change 190–192

Kuhn, Thomas S. 182

Kuypers, Leah M. 146–147

least restrictive environment (LRE) 6, 11, 18, 126

legislative foundation, history 5–16; 1960s–1970s 5; 1973, Rehabilitation Act, Section 504 / 504 Plans 16, **16**, 74–75, 182; 1974, Family Educational Rights and Privacy Act (FERPA) 15–16; 1975, Education for All Handicapped Children Act (EHA) 6–7; 1990/2004, Individuals with Disabilities Education Act (IDEA) 6–12 (*see also under own heading*); 1996, Health Insurance and Portability and Accountability Act (HIPAA) 15–16; 2015, Every Student Succeeds Act (ESSA) 3, 13–15, **15**, 70 (*see also* multi-tiered system of supports (MTSS)); pre-1960 5

legislative foundation, occupational therapy as related service 16–27; definition 16; IDEA, 1990/2004 6–7, 11, 16–17; inclusive education 18, 21–25; practitioners, qualification requirements 17; practitioners, scope of practice 17–18; Universal design for learning (UDL) 19–21, 24, 43, 45, 83, 134, 180

Likert scales 103, 161, 164, 166

Mailloux, Z. 122, **123**

Medicaid 15, 16, 24, 62, 185

modulation and modulation disorders, sensory processing 34, 43, 47, 82, 85–86, **86**, 105

motor planning 37, 39, *40*, **73**, *110*

MTSS, Tier 1 (school, classroom) 14, **15**, 151–153, 212–213; Alert Program, alertness levels impact 117, 146; ASI guidance and application 124–125; discharge planning 174; EHP guidance and application 125–126; fidelity, interventions 200; free play support 145; goal setting 127, 128–129; intervention development considerations 70–71, 117; intervention examples 59; intervention outcomes evaluation 162, 163; intervention targets 14, **57**, 58–59; occupational performance evaluation 97, 105; occupational therapist's role 51, 56, 64, 70, 181, 184–186, *187–188*, 193–194, 196, 214; OTPF-4 application **57**;

outcome evaluation 162; PEO model guidance and application 59, 122–124, **123**, 129; progress monitoring 65, 111; sensory environment interventions, designing and modifications 51, 59–60, 63, 68, 70, 97, 122, 134–136, 150–151, *152*; Sensory Ladders program 149; sensory support 134–136; Zones of Regulation curriculum 147, 148

MTSS, Tier 2 (group level) 14–15, **15**, 60–61, 151–153, 215–217; Alert Program, alertness levels impact 146; ASI guidance and application 124, 125; discharge planning 174–175; EHP guidance and application 125, 126; fidelity, interventions 200; goal setting 127, 128, 129, 136; intervention development considerations 72–73, **73**; intervention targets 14, 14–15, 50–51, **57**, 60–61; interventions need prevalence 53; occupational performance evaluation 97, 105; occupational therapist's role, school integration 51, 56, 64, 117, 136, 171, 181, 184–186, *187–190*, 196, 202, 206, 217; occupational therapist's role 51; OTPF-4 application **57**; PEO model guidance and application 122–124, **123**; progress monitoring 65, 111; sensory environment interventions, designing and modifications 60, 97, 117, 122, 134–136, 151–153, **153**; Sensory Ladders program 149; Tier 2/3 blending 61, *62*; Zones of Regulation curriculum 148

MTSS, Tier 3 (individual) 62–63, 217–218; ASI guidance and application 124, 125; discharge planning 174–175, 218, 218–219; evaluation (eligibility, performance, outcome) 80, *81*, 104, 105, 158; intervention targets and development 15, **57**, 62, 74–75; occupational therapist's role, school integration 3, 51, 175, 181, 185, 195, 217–218, 220; sensory environment, designing and modifications 117; sensory environment interventions, designing and modifications 73, 117; Tier 2/3 blending 61, *62*, 216; *see also* Individualized Education Plan (IEP)

multidisciplinary teams 179–202; attitudinal barriers 192–193; caseload vs workload 183–184; change management (Knoster Model application) 191–192; client approach differences 193; collective responsibility 196; communication methods 193; evaluation 81, *81*, 86; interprofessional model 193–194; occupational therapist-classroom teacher cooperation 2; organizational support 184–185; relationship forming, schoolwide 194–195; sensory support needs and competency requirements 179–180; time and resource needs negotiations (Tier 1, 2) 185–187, *187–189*, 190; time restrictions and collaborative advocacy 144, 185–190, 195–196; training school personnel, teachers 24, 45, 47, 64, 168–170, *188–189*, 191, 196–200, 212–213, 216

Multi-Tiered System of Supports and Occupational Therapy and Sensory Needs (MTSS) 14–15, **15**, 50–75; evidence-based interventions 14; interprofessional team nature 14; legislative foundation (ESSA, 2015) 13, 50; neuro-affirming vs deficit approach 165; occupational therapist's role 51; OTPF-4 to MTSS level application 56–57, **57**; progress monitoring 52, 65–68, *67*, **68**, 70, 72 (*see also under own heading*); progress monitoring, systematic data collection 14; roots, initiating base experiences 1–3; as RTI model extension 13, 14, 50, 175, *188–189*; sense making process 67–70, 74; tier level decisions, needs assessment 14, 14–15, **15**, 51, **57**, 70, 78 (*see also* need assessment); tier system 13, 14–15, **15** (*see also* MTSS, Tiers 1/2/3); universal screening 14, **15**, 52, 53–56, **55**, 60, 72, 163–164, 188–189; universal screening in MTSS 14, **15**, 52, 53–56, **55**, 60, 72, 163–164, 188–189

neuro-affirming approaches, learning 20–21, 165

neurodiverse students 19, 20–21, 45, 165

neurodiversity-affirming education, as UDL component 20–21, 45

No Child Left Behind Act (2002) 12
norm-referenced assessments 157–158

observations: checklist 54, *55*; criterion-
referenced assessments 158; fidelity
172, 200, 213; informal data source **68**,
87; observer report 162; occupational
performance 97–100, **98**, 99–*100*, *99*;
occupational profiles 93; Structured
Observations of Sensory Integration-
Motor (SOSI-M) 82–83, **88**, 162; task–
activity transition 88–90, **89**
occupational history gathering 61, **95–96**,
95, 97
occupational performance analysis 78, 86,
97–106; direct assessment 105–106;
interviews, focus groups 87, 94–95, 97,
100–102, 103, *103*, 106; observations
97–100 (*see also under own heading*);
as part of the evaluation process 78, 97,
108–109; questionnaires 104–105, **104**
(*see also under own heading*); surveys
103–104
occupational profiles 78–79, 93–95,
95–96, **95**, 97
occupational therapy as related service;
see related service, occupational
therapy as
Occupational therapy practice framework:
Domain and process –Fourth edition
(OTPF-4) 54, 56–57, **57**, 59, 61, 85, 93,
105, 170, 208
olfactory sensory system, environment,
stimulation/activities 22, 33, **37**,
44, **131**
outcomes 160–164; distal 85, 90–93, **91**,
92, 106, 108, 109, **123**, 168; evaluation
(*see* intervention outcome evaluation);
performance-based 161–162; program
outcomes 162–164; proximal 85–87,
90–91, 106, 108–109, 109, **123**, 168;
reporting (self, by proxy, observer)
161, 162

Parham, Diane **42**, 43
Participation and Sensory Environment
Questionnaire–Teacher Version
(PSEQ–TV) 91–93, *92*, **104**
Person-Environment-Occupation, PEO
model 21, 59, 122–123, 126, 148

positive behavior interventions and
support (PBI&S) plan 166–167, 177
Positive Behavioral Support (PBS) 13
postural control, postural disorders 32, 33,
36, **42**, 51, **88**, *110*
postural sensorimotor disorders 36
predictive validity, assessment
measures 160
preference, sensory 63, *64*, 196, 208–209,
212, 216
program outcomes 162–164
progress monitoring *23*, 24, 61, 167–176;
Ayre Sensory Integration® (ASI) 122,
123; case study (Anabelle, progress
monitoring, support adaptation) *176*;
concept, definition 52; data (collection,
quality, use) 52, 65–67, 127, 167–
168, *169*, 170–174 (*see also under
own heading*); Ecology of Human
Performance (EHP) 126; Every Student
Succeeds Act (ESSA, 2015) 13;
fidelity, interventions 41–43, **42**, 124,
168–170, *169*, 172–173, 197, 200–201,
213; Knoster's Model for Managing
Complex Change 191; Multi-Tiered
System of Supports (MTSS) 15,
52, 65–68, 84, 111, 127–129, 156,
167–171, 200, 218; purpose of 167;
Response to Intervention (RTI) 13,
14; sense making process 67–70, 74;
steps 65–68, *67*, **68**, 168, *169*; universal
screening 54, 163–164; *see also* data,
collection and quality
proprioceptive sensory systems 32, **45**,
91, **131**, 137–139
proximal outcomes 85–87, 90–91, 106,
108–109, 109, **123**, 168
psychometric assessment properties 112,
157, 158–160, 163, 177

questionnaires 104–108, **104**, 106–107,
111–112, 161; child's perspective
106–108, *107–108*; Classroom
Sensory Environment Assessment
(C-SEA) **104**; informal 104–105;
Participation and Sensory Environment
Questionnaire–Teacher Version
(PSEQ–TV) 91–93, *92*, **104**; sample,
sensory and satisfaction *107–108*;
Sensory and Satisfaction Questionnaire

107, *107–108*, 161; Sensory Processing Measure-2 (SPM-2) 82–83, **86**, **104**, 161; Sensory Profile 2 (SP2) **86**, 87, **104**, 161; standardized 104, **104**

reactivity and modulation, sensory processing 34–36; assessment, evaluation 81–83, 85–86, **86**, 90, 105, 109, 111–112, 116; hyperreactivity 35, 39, 90, 116, 119–120, 130, 132, 151–152, 208, 215; hyporeactivity 35, 36, 38–39, 90, 116, 130, 132, 215; modulation and modulation disorders 34, 43, 47, 82, 85–86, **86**, 105; sensory defensiveness / experience avoidance 35

related service, occupational therapy 16–27; definition, concept 16, 125; inclusive education 18, 21–25 (*see also under own heading*); legislative foundation (IDEA, 1990/2004) 6–7, 11, 16–17; practitioners, qualification requirements 17; practitioners, scope of practice 17–18, 51, 82, 125, 158, 168; related service vs eligibility category 158; Universal design for learning (UDL) 19–21, 24, 43, 45, 83, 134, 180

reliability: assessment measures 81, 91, 158, 159; clinical utility 160; outcome measure types 159

representation as UDL component 20

Response to Intervention (RTI) 13, 14, 50, 175, *188–189*

Schaaf, R. C. 122, **123**

school-based sensory techniques 43, **44**; *see also* sensory-based interventions (SBIs)

Section 504, Rehabilitation Act (1973) / 504 Plan 16, **16**, 74–75, 182

sensorimotor disorders 32, 34, 36–38, **37**, 52–53

Sensory and Satisfaction Questionnaire 107, *107–108*, 161

sensory bins 140, 206, 215

sensory defensiveness / experience avoidance 35

sensory environment 43–46, 124–125; as ASI component **42**; Classroom Sensory Environment Assessment (C-SEA) **104**;

inclusive education settings 18–19, 21–22; least restrictive environment (LRE) 6, 11, 18, 126; Person-Environment-Occupation, PEO model 21, 59, 122–123, 126, 148; sensory processing, impact 30–31, 43, 45, 53; sensory systems, stimuli and interaction (*see* sensory systems); universal design for learning (UDL) 19; universal screening 54, *55*

sensory environment, assessment/ evaluation: criteria 22; intervention outcomes 85–87, **85**, 172, 173; observations (*see under own heading*); occupational performance impact 97–99, 109, 110–111; occupational therapist's roles 22, 82; Participation and Sensory Environment Questionnaire–Teacher Version (PSEQ–TV) 91–93, *92*, **104**; requirement for 83–84; Structured Observations of Sensory Integration-Motor (SOSI-M) 82–83, **88**, 162; transitions, task–activity 88–90, **89**

sensory environment, designing and modifications 219; data-driven decision-making (DDDM) 70, 122, 123; educator, teacher training 45, 219; flexibility, adaptability 45, 46; free play opportunities 142, 144; MTSS Tier 1 (school, classroom) 51, 59–60, 63, 68, 70, 97, 122, 134–136, 150–151, *152*; MTSS Tier 2 (small groups, home) 60, 97, 117, 122, 134–136, 151–153, **153**; MTSS Tier 3 (individual) 73, 117; occupational therapist as expert and lead 83, 92–93, 144, 167; PEO model 122–123, 126, 148; tactile 119–120, **131**, 133–134, *135*; techniques 43–47; visual 22, 33, 38, **44**, 45–46, **91**, **131**, 142

sensory integration and processing 30–48; alertness levels impact 36, 117–119, **119–120**, 146–147, 149, *197*; case study (Anthony, sensory processing differences) *39–41*; definition 30; and learning 38–39, *39–41*; modulation and reactivity (*see* reactivity and modulation, sensory processing); personal nature, individual variations

of 30, 31; process 30–31, 34–36;
processing dysfunction and disorders
31, 47; sensorimotor disorders 32, 34,
36–38, **37**; sensory systems function
(*see under own heading*); sensory-
based interventions 43, **44**; theory (A.
Jean Ayres) 30–33, 41–43, 47, 61 (*see
also* Ayre Sensory Integration® (ASI))
sensory integration therapy 41; *see also*
Ayre Sensory Integration® (ASI)
sensory interventions: vs ASI 124–125;
sensory environmental modifications
22, 43–47, 59, 83, 92, 117, 130–132,
132, 134–135, 219; sensory techniques
41, 43, **44**, 124–125, 198, 214–215,
219; sensory-based interventions (SBIs)
31, 41–43, 47, 51, 74, 83–84, 124–125;
teacher training and coaching 47
Sensory Ladders 148–149, *150*
sensory memory 35
Sensory Processing Measure-2 (SPM-2)
82–83, **86**, **104**, 161
Sensory Profile 2 (SP2) **86**, 87, **104**, 161
sensory systems 31–34, **34**, **37**, 47;
assessment (Ayres Sensory Integration)
116, 124; associated activities 136–142;
auditory 33, 38, **44**, 45–46, **91**, **131**,
142; body awareness 32; cognitive
regulation programs 146–150; distance
33; environment modification 45,
131; free play 142; gustatory 34, **37**;
interoception 34, **37**; and learning
38–39; movement 118; olfactory
22, 33, **37**, **44**, **131**; proprioceptive
32, **45**, **91**, **131**, 137–139; and
sensory input principles **37**; sensory
processing in 90, **91**, 109, **109**;
sensory-based intervention impact
43, **44–45**; somatosensory 32; tactile
(somatosensory) 32, **44**, **91**, 120, **131**,
139–140, *141*; vestibular 22, 32–33, 36,
44, **91**, *110–111*, **131**, 136–137, 144;
visual 33, 38, **44**, 45–46, **91**, **131**, 142
sensory threshold *110*, *111*, 116–117,
119, 142
sensory-based interventions (SBIs) 31,
41–43, 47, 51, 74, 83–84, 124–125
Shellenberger, Shelly 146
Short Child Occupational Profile
(SCOPE) 162
SMART goal 111
Smith, Kath 148–149

social and emotional learning (SEL)
curriculum 145, 214–215
Social Thinking curriculum 146–147
somatosensory system, environment,
stimulation/activities 32, 36, **44**, **91**,
110, 120, **131**, 139–140, *141*
Stansberry, A. *107–108*
strength-based intervention approaches
14, 21, 58, 105, 112, 124, 165, 196
Structured Observations of Sensory
Integration-Motor (SOSI-M) 82–83,
88, 162
student-centered practices, interventions
21, 164–166
surveys 103–104, 164

tactile input types 119–120
tactile sensory system, environment,
stimulation/activities 32, 34, **44**, 61, **91**,
119–120, **131**, 139–140, *141*
task–activity transition 88–90, **89**
teach-back method 197, 198
test-retest reliability 159
The Alert Program 47, 146, 147, 212
The Structure of Scientific Revolutions
(Kuhn) 182
training school personnel, teachers 24,
45, 47, 64, 168–170, *188–189*, 191,
196–200, 212–213, 216
Two Truths and a Lie, game **96**

Universal design for learning (UDL)
19–21, 24, 43, 45, 83, 134, 180
universal screening, MTSS 14, **15**, 52,
53–56, **55**, 60, 72, 163–164, 188–189

validity, assessment measures 81, 91, 158,
159–160
vestibular sensory system, environment,
stimulation/activities 22, 32–33, 36, **44**,
91, *110–111*, **131**, 136–137, 144
visual sensory system, environment,
stimulation/activities 22, 33, 38, **44**,
45–46, **91**, **131**, 142

Weick, Karl E. 68
weighted items 134, *134*, *135*, **151**, *209*, *211*
Whiting, C. C. 43
Williams, Mary Sue 146

Zones of Regulation 146–148, *148*,
176, 212